Springer Series on the Teaching of Nursing

Diane O. McGivern, RN, PhD, FAAN, Series Editor
New York University Division of Nursing

Advisory Board: Ellen Baer, PhD, RN, FAAN; Carla Mariano, EdD, RN; Janet A. Rodgers, PhD, RN, FAAN; Alice Adam Young, PhD, RN

Joyce E. (Beebe) Thompson, RN, CNM, DrPH, FAAN, FACNM, is Professor and Associate Dean for Graduate and Professional Studies at the University of Pennsylvania School of Nursing in Philadelphia. A certified nurse-midwife since 1966, Dr. Thompson has taught midwifery in certificate and master's programs since 1971. She also teaches ethics and leadership development, and directs the Teacher Education Program at the University of Pennsylvania School of Nursing. She has taught and consulted in nursing, midwifery, Safe Motherhood, and ethics in South America and East-Central Africa. She is the primary drafter of the essential competencies in midwifery practice that are being field-tested for use globally by the International Confederation of Midwives. A teacher of teachers, Dr. Thompson is committed to extending the influence and effectiveness of nurses and midwives throughout the world, beginning with high quality education.

Rose M. Kershbaumer, RN, CNM, MSN, EdD, Medical Mission Sister, is Assistant to the Director of the World Health Organization (WHO) Collaborating Center for Nursing and Midwifery Leadership, University of Pennsylvania School of Nursing, and Co-Director and teacher in the Teacher Education Program. She received her RN from Jefferson Medical College Hospital School of Nursing and her CNM from Catholic Maternity Institute in Santa Fe, New Mexico. Her BSN and MSN are from the University of Pennsylvania in Philadelphia, and she gained her EdD from Teachers College, Columbia University. Dr. Kershbaumer has extensive experience as a nurse-midwife in sub-Saharan Africa and as a WHO Nurse Educator and Coordinator in the Africa Region.

Mary Ann Krisman-Scott, RN, PhD, FNP, is a Family Nurse Practitioner and received her BSN from Catholic University in Washington, DC and her MSN and PhD from the University of Pennsylvania. She has taught in the Teacher Education program since its inception and in the Nurse Practitioner program at the University of Pennsylvania and coordinated the Pediatric Nurse Practitioner Program at the University of Hawaii. She currently coordinates the Pediatric Nurse Practitioner Program at the University of South Florida. Her clinical practice has focused on the care of adolescents and women's health care.

EDUCATING ADVANCED PRACTICE NURSES AND MIDWIVES

FROM PRACTICE TO TEACHING

Joyce E. Thompson, RN, CNM, Dr.PH, FAAN, FACNM

Rose M. Kershbaumer, MMS, RN, CNM, MSN, EdD

Mary Ann Krisman-Scott, RN, PhD, FNP

 Springer Series on the Teaching of Nursing

Springer Publishing Company, Inc.
536 Broadway
New York, NY 10012-3955

Acquisitions Editor: Sheri W. Sussman
Production Editor: Jeanne Libby
Cover design by Susan Hauley

01 02 03 04 05/5 4 3 2 1

Library of Congress Cataloging-in-Publication Data

Thompson, Joyce Beebe.
  Educating advanced practice nurses and midwives : from practice to teaching / Joyce E. Thompson, Rose M. Kershbaumer, Mary Ann Krisman-Scott.
    p. cm.
  Includes bibliographical references and index.
  ISBN 0-8261-1437-7
  1. Nurse practitioners—Study and teaching. 2. Midwifery—Study and teaching.
I. Kershbaumer, Rose M. II. Krisman-Scott, Mary Ann. III. Title.
[DNLM: 1. Education, Nursing—methods—Teaching. 2. Midwifery—education—Teaching.
WY 18 T473e 2001]
RT82.8.T475 2001
610.73'06'92—dc21

                                            2001020929

Printed in Canada by Tri-Graphics, Inc.

This text is dedicated to the loving memory of
Rev. Dr. Henry O. Thompson, MDiv, PhD
Mentor, Teacher, Friend, Husband

Contents

Contents

Contributor

Michele A. Goldfarb, Esq.
Director, Office of Student Conduct
University of Pennsylvania
Philadelphia, Pennsylvania

Foreword

As the professions of nursing and midwifery move into the rapidly changing health and illness care systems of the 21st century, so must the education of nurses and midwives. Faculty who prepare the nurses and midwives for the future are required to not only have the current best knowledge in their content area, but must also know how to generate new knowledge and disseminate it through writing and teaching others. While much of the preparation of faculty today has a strong focus on research, very little is offered to help the potential faculty member learn the education role. Similarly, the preparation of clinicians has a strong focus on practice with little, if any, content on how to teach others to do what they do. This book is a major contribution to all faculty, staff, clinicians, and preceptors who select the vital and exciting role of teacher.

As a young nurse faculty member many years ago, I found myself looking for help in my teaching role. I had the good fortune to come upon a most helpful book, *The Art of Clinical Instruction*, by Lillian Sholtis and Jane Bragdon.* The book soon became a well-used resource that I consulted for guidance on all aspects of curriculum and instruction.

Drs. Joyce Beebe Thompson, Rose Kershbaumer, and Mary Ann Krisman Scott nearly a decade ago identified the serious need to prepare teachers of advanced practice nurses and midwives. They designed and implemented a contemporary educational program for faculty and clinicians who wish to become expert teachers. This book is a result of that successful Teacher Education Program targeting faculty for the 21st century. The authors' combined decades of teaching and clinical experience offer very useful philosophical, theoretical, and practical support for all aspects of teaching in a health discipline. This new text will quickly become an expert reference for both the novice and experienced teacher

---

*Sholtis, L. S., & J.S. Bragdon (1961). *The Art of Clinical Instruction*. Philadelphia: J. B. Lipincott Company.

in today's Schools of Nursing, other health professional schools, and their partner clinical agencies.

Norma M. Lang, PhD, RN, FAAN, FRCN
Former Margaret Bond Simon Dean
Lillian S. Brunner Professor of Medical Surgical Nursing
University of Pennsylvania
School of Nursing
Philadelphia, Pennsylvania
USA

Preface

You cannot teach a man anything; you can only help him find it within himself.

—Galileo

The truly artistic teacher of adults . . . conscientiously suppresses his own compulsion to teach what he knows his students ought to learn in favor of helping his students learn for themselves what they want to learn.

—Knowles, 1970

This text has been written as a guide to new teachers of advanced practice nurses (APNs) and midwives, who are themselves making the transition from clinicians to educators.

VALUES AND BELIEFS ABOUT TEACHING AND LEARNING

Any book on teaching must address the values and beliefs of its authors, since teaching is about entering the minds and lives of the learner. Teachers and teaching enter not only the psychomotor and cognitive domains of learning, but also the affective domain. We share the belief that if values are not taught, they will be caught. As experienced teachers, we prefer to clearly expose our own values related to teaching and learning as we also teach values related to midwifery and advanced practice nursing to others. It is therefore important that any reader and user of this text understand the values and beliefs shared by the authors. The philosophy of the authors sets the tone for our success in teaching and learning and clearly articulates some of the beliefs and values that we hold as teachers. Our philosophy of teaching is:

Learning is fun, and teaching fulfills many hopes and dreams for those who are willing and eager to help others learn. In keeping with the ideas of Gilbert Highet, the best of teaching and learning occurs when teaching "stops being the mere transmission of information and becomes the joint enterprise of a group of friendly human beings who like using their brains" (Highet, 1950, p. 153). The authors believe that as we think, we practice. Likewise, as we teach, we must always be mindful of the relationship between thinking and practice.

We believe that teaching adults requires a different approach than that used when teaching children. Adults (professional nurses) are self-motivated, goal-directed, and learn best in situations where they can immediately apply what they are learning. Adults also learn what they think is useful in attaining their professional goals, and are willing and able to be responsible for their own learning. We also believe that learning is a life-long process. The primary goal of teaching, therefore, is to help others learn.

We believe that understanding how people learn is first and foremost the foundation for effective teaching. When working with adults, each principle of learning should be matched to a corresponding principle of teaching. Adults, moreover, have experienced many learning opportunities in their life, and have developed a variety of patterns of learning. Therefore, teaching adults requires a variety of approaches along with the exquisite use of self in interaction and communication with others.

The core of teaching others to teach includes helping individuals acquire the skills to teach critical thinking, clinical judgment, and accountability for decisions made in the roles of nurse-midwife and nurse practitioner. We believe that each teacher must be a role model of these essential skills and be able to teach both the art and the science of professional practice.

DECISIONS NEEDED BEFORE TEACHING

There are many aspects of teaching in a clinical discipline that are similar to those of any discipline. However, the presence of both a health professional learner and a patient in the teacher-learner equation adds a note of complexity that does not exist in the teaching of the basic sciences, philosophy, or religion. Most teachers of advanced practice nursing and midwifery have a strong clinical base from which to promote learning these clinical roles. Therefore, these teachers have been teaching patients and families well before thinking about teaching others to do what they do as clinicians. Teaching patients is one of the hallmarks of the nursing and midwifery models of care, based on the belief that health promotion begins with knowledge shared with the recipients of care so that they can take action to keep themselves as healthy as possible. Learning about the teaching role of the health professional is an integral component of one's advanced preparation in nursing and midwifery. Individual and group educational strategies are reinforced with practice. All teaching, as well as practice efforts, is based on exquisite communication skills.

Decisions needed before taking on the teaching role include what will be taught, to whom, where, when, and how. We start from the premise that the *what* of teaching is advanced practice nursing and midwifery, the *who* are those adults choosing these health professional roles, and the *where* includes both classroom and clinical environments within the context of a university-based educational program. *When* you teach specific content and *how* that content will be taught depends in large measure on the level of the learner. For example, teachers make decisions about what content will come first in the curriculum, moving from the simple to the complex. Likewise, expectations for performance of a first level learner are quite different from expectations of a learner about to complete an educational program. These decisions reflect the preparation of the teacher in the philosophy of teaching and learning, learning theory, curriculum development, and teaching and evaluation methods. Both the science and art of teaching are essential to effective learning.

ORGANIZATION OF THE TEXT

This text is organized to follow the authors' beliefs, values, and experience in preparing for the teaching role. The first chapter provides the historical foundations and lessons learned about nurse practitioner and midwifery education that set the stage for current approaches to preparing advanced practice nurses and midwives. Since the text is devoted to providing the foundation for teaching and the major transition of clinician to teacher, the second chapter reviews some of the relevant transition theory in nursing. Chapters 3 and 4 provide the ethical and philosophical foundations for teaching health professionals, and chapter 5 highlights the importance of critical thinking in advanced practice nursing and midwifery education and practice. Chapter 6 reviews the various influences on teaching and learning brought to the educational milieu by teachers and learners.

Chapters 7 through 12 concentrate on the basics of "how" to prepare for and carry out the teaching role in classroom and clinical settings. This includes the theoretical foundations of human learning, principles that guide the teacher in helping APNs and nurse-midwives acquire the requisite theory for their professional discipline, curriculum development, and strategies to implement the curriculum. The final three chapters deal with the more administrative aspects of teaching in an advanced practice discipline, including setting up and maintaining clinical sites, academic responsibilities, and legal aspects of teaching.

The central focuses of this text are to help the teacher develop an understanding of: how adults learn, APN and midwifery curricula, and how to foster learning of the advanced practice nursing and midwifery roles. Each chapter begins with a statement of outcomes and ends with several questions for reflection and study. Some tools are included as examples along with suggested exercises for testing out the content presented in the chapter. References and selected bibliographic citations are included for the reader who wishes to read in more detail selected concepts discussed in the text.

The primary motivation for writing this text came from several years of experience and success in teaching others how to teach advanced practice nurses and midwives. The authors designed, implemented, and continue to evaluate their efforts in the Teacher Education Program at the University of Pennsylvania School of Nursing. While it is nearly impossible to put the enthusiasm and excitement of direct contact with these adults learners on the pages of this text, our current teacher-learners and graduates continue to inspire us to learn even more about teaching and learning. We hope that you will also find this teaching role as exciting, challenging, and rewarding as we do.

J. E. THOMPSON,
R. M. KERSHBAUMER,
AND M. A. KRISMAN-SCOTT

CHAPTER 1

A Brief History of Midwifery and Nurse Practitioner Education in the United States

> What experience and history teach is this—that people and governments never have learned anything from history, or acted on principles deduced from it.
>
> — Hegel, *Werke*

SUGGESTED OUTCOMES FOR THIS CHAPTER

At the end of this chapter, the reader will be able to

1. describe key factors that have led to the development of the disciplines of midwifery and nurse-midwifery in the United States,
2. describe the era and events that led to and supported the development of nurse practitioners in the United States, and
3. define recurring themes from history that influence and direct advanced practice nursing and midwifery education today.

INTRODUCTION

The authors are firm believers in the value of understanding history, and the lessons that one can learn from the study of history that help to inform what is happening today and what the possibilities may be for tomorrow. Lynaugh (1991) notes that history allows us to do what science prohibits; that is, history explores unique events in unique lives rather than the laws of science based on commonalities of events and responses. The exploration of the unique historical events that have led to present-day education and practice in midwifery and advanced practice nursing tells us much about the struggles, decisions, and forward thinking of our foremothers. Recurring themes arise in the midwifery to nurse-midwifery and nurse practitioner movements in the United States. If we are to be wise learners as teachers, we need to understand where our profession has come from, what influenced its development, and what we can learn that will help guide the professions in the future; that is, how we should design the education of practitioners for tomorrow's demands. This chapter addresses some of these issues briefly, but is only the beginning in presenting the history and interpretation of midwifery and the nurse practitioner movement in the United States. Original sources are included in the bibliography for your continued study and reflection, and you are strongly encouraged to do this before embarking on your teaching career.

HISTORY OF MIDWIFERY AND NURSE-MIDWIFERY

The history of midwifery is as ancient as men and women themselves. From the earliest times, women have been with women during childbirth. In fact, the earliest recorded information about midwives appears in the Bible, Genesis 35:17, "And it came to pass, when she was in hard labour, that the midwife said unto her, 'Fear not . . . ' " This chapter will not attempt to trace the long history and traditions of midwifery from the beginnings of the human race. It will focus on the development and practice of midwifery in the United States in the early 20th century and the evolution to the present-day nurse-midwife. As noted by Burst (1991), nurse-midwifery "is an ancient profession reborn in contemporary society."

Immigrant and Granny Midwives

Midwifery as a distinct discipline or profession has many historical roots that reflect its practitioners' commitment to be "with woman" wherever she resides, in whatever condition she finds herself, and to be with the woman's family and support systems during childbirth. The basis for the modern profession of nurse-midwifery in the United States is firmly grounded in the traditions of safe, satisfying, and effective practice of midwives who migrated to this country, mostly from Europe and Africa, in order to care for the pregnant women in their ethnic groups (Ulrich, 1990; Walsh, 1991). These immigrant and granny or "grand" midwives held the future of this wonderful nation in their hands with each birth attended, and their record of safety and healthy outcomes for mothers and newborns far exceeded the record of physicians who were attending births at the beginning of the 20th century (Walsh, 1991; Wertz & Wertz, 1977).

Struggles, Conflicts, and Controversies

The history of midwifery in the United States in the early 1900s was filled with struggles, conflicts, and controversies (Burst, 1991). Even though midwives had a long tradition of success in the practice of midwifery, their very success caused physicians and nurses to attack them. These attacks came primarily out of jealousy over the midwife's respected role within the community where she lived and the fact that physicians began to compete with midwives for attendance at birth. This was especially true as the medical profession became strong and the specialty of obstetrics evolved. Burst (1991) notes that obstetricians, in their struggle for recognition and status, had to deem pregnancy a pathological condition that needed hospitals and physicians. They could not admit that pregnancy was normal and could be safely attended by such a "simple" person as the often untrained, barely literate midwife. Even after midwifery education was standardized in the United States, competition for control of pregnancy and birth by physicians continued (Varney, 1997). One of the saddest examples of the medical establishment using vulnerable childbearing women as political pawns in interprofessional rivalry was the refusal of the California Medical Society to allow Armentia Jarrett, Certified Nurse-Midwife, to continue midwifery care in Madera County in the 1960s. When nurse-midwives were forced to cease giving care to these vulnerable women, there was a dramatic increase in preterm births and neonatal deaths (Levy, Wilkinson, & Marine, 1971).

Early immigrant midwives in the United States suffered from a lack of standardized midwifery curricula (Rooks, 1997), had little or no means of communicating with one another or updating their knowledge base (Burst, 1991), and many lacked legal recognition (Rooks, 1997; Varney, 1997) or status in society—especially in the rural south (Robinson, 1984). Burst (1991) comments that the history of midwifery in the United States is closely intertwined with the history of women and their lack of status within any policy making body. The "midwife problem" surfaced amid debates as to whether all midwives should be abolished or whether midwives should be properly educated and supervised (controlled) in their practice—either by physicians or public health nurses. As Varney (1997) summarizes, those in favor of midwives recognized that the poor showing of the U.S. in maternal and infant mortality and morbidity could not be addressed solely by physicians and that a properly trained, licensed, and supervised midwife could provide valuable services to childbearing women. Those opposed to having any midwife attending birth "feared the status [that] midwives would gain if they achieved legal recognition" (Varney, 1997, p. 7). This fear of the success of the midwives in keeping women healthy led to professional rivalry that continued well into the second half of the 20th century. Early schools established to provide midwifery training as mandated by legislation included the Bellevue School of Midwifery (1911–1935) in New York City and the Preston Retreat Hospital in Philadelphia (1923–1930). These schools were established to instruct indigenous midwives (Varney, 1997). The Shepherd-Towner Act of 1921 included a provision for using public health nurses to train and supervise untrained midwives in an effort to enhance prenatal care as well as birth care (Thompson, Walsh, & Merkatz, 1990). These schools were short-lived as childbearing care steadily improved and those in power felt there was no longer a need to train midwives. The specialty of obstetrics was growing, and the midwives were seen as no longer necessary.

Emergence of the Nurse-Midwife

In 1925, about the same time that immigrant and granny midwives were being forced out of practice or giving it up as more and more women chose the hospital setting—where midwives were not allowed (Litoff, 1978; Rooks, 1997), nurse-midwives from Europe were introduced into Frontier Nursing Service (FNS) in Hyden, Kentucky, by Mary Breckinridge. Her goal was to provide health care for those living in the rural mountains and hollers of Kentucky—the vulnerable, the poor, the forgotten (Breckinridge, 1952). The nurse-midwife of the 21st century is still providing care following this commitment to vulnerable populations of women and the midwifery model of care established at FNS. The work of the FNS public health nurses and nurse-midwives in promoting the health of families and childbearing women is legendary, with outcome statistics far better than the national averages for many decades (Metropolitan Life, 1958).

Safety and Efficacy of Nurse-Midwifery Practice

Many studies on the safety and effectiveness of nurse-midwifery practice since the early days of Frontier Nursing Service have repeatedly demonstrated the success of nurse-midwives in promoting the health of women and newborns, and in preventing both morbidity and mortality (Thompson, J. E., 1986). Nurse-midwives have kept detailed statistics on their practice outcomes since the first service began in 1925 (Metropolitan Life, 1958). With a commitment to safe care, outcome statistics have been the predominant method of assessing the safety of nurse-midwifery practice over the years, with more recent studies focusing on both process and outcome measures of the quality of care provided (Thompson,

J. E., 1986). The significance of early and ongoing evaluative studies reinforce that well-prepared nurse-midwives provide childbearing care both in and out of hospital that is not only as good as, but at times, better than that offered by medical personnel, controlling for the risk conditions of the pregnant women (Rooks et al., 1989). In addition to the safety of midwifery care, measures of satisfaction are often greater with nurse-midwives than with other medical personnel (Record & Cohen, 1972; Thompson, 1981). In 1986, the Office of Technology Assessment (OTA) studied care given by nurse practitioners, physician assistants, and certified nurse-midwives (CNMs) and affirmed the high quality, safety, and effectiveness of that care (OTA, 1986). This was again reaffirmed by the American Nurses Association (ANA) in 1993 with a meta-analysis of the process of care, clinical outcomes, and cost effectiveness of nurses in primary care roles including nurse practitioners and nurse-midwives (ANA, 1993). Nurse-midwives have a more than 75-year history of providing safe, satisfying, and cost-quality efficient care for women and their families. The model of midwifery care that is built upon respect for human dignity and self-worth, promotes health, empowers women and families, and makes a difference in the health of any nation is also characterized by educating women/families so that they can become active and knowledgeable participants in their own health care decisions, while ever mindful of the need for safety (Thompson, Oakley, Burke, Jay, & Conklin, 1989). Strong educational preparation has been and continues to be essential to becoming safe, effective, and caring clinicians.

Schools of Nurse-Midwifery

The first nurse-midwifery education program was established in New York City in 1932. It was called the Lobenstine Midwifery School, and then became Maternity Center Association's (MCA) School of Nurse-Midwifery (MCA, 1955). Rose McNaught, a public health nurse educated in midwifery in London, was loaned from FNS to begin the school, with Hattie Hemschemeyer, a public health nurse educator, as the Director (Shoemaker, 1947; Varney, 1997). From 1932 to 1958, the Maternity Center Association School of Nurse-Midwifery provided instruction in midwifery at the Center with clinical experience in the clinic and births primarily in the home. In 1958, MCA joined together with Downstate Medical Center, State University of New York, Brooklyn, and the faculty and students began to provide hospital-based midwifery services. This entry into the hospital setting was facilitated by Dr. Louis Hellman, director of the department of obstetrics and gynecology. Dr. Hellman was a strong supporter of nurse-midwifery and was nearly censored by the OB/GYN society for his open valuing of the nurse-midwife as a vital partner in the care of childbearing women (Burst, 1991). In 1939, FNS began educating nurse-midwives in the Frontier Graduate School of Midwifery, and in 1945, the Medical Mission Sisters established the Catholic Maternity Institute (CMI) School of Nurse-Midwifery in Santa Fe, New Mexico. The nurse-midwives and students attended births in the home until 1953, when most of those requesting home birth were now attended in the first freestanding birth center in the U.S. called, 'La Casita' (CMI, 1994).

Early educational programs in nurse-midwifery served poor, rural, and inner-city women, with births in homes or birth centers. They had no university affiliation even though the nurse-midwifery leaders believed that midwifery education belonged in the university setting (Burst, 1991). In 1947, the first university affiliation was established between Catholic University of America (CUA) and the Catholic Maternity Institute (CMI). The graduates received their master's degree from CUA and their midwifery preparation from CMI. The first master's program in maternity nursing and nurse-midwifery (MSN) located totally within a university was at Columbia University School of Nursing, which admitted its first students in 1955. Yale University followed in 1956, New York Medical College in 1963, and the University of Utah in 1965.

Current nurse-midwifery educational programs in the United States have followed closely the curriculum in midwifery imported from Europe, especially the United Kingdom, where midwifery education and practice has been very strong and well respected for over a century (Rooks, 1997). The great majority of these programs were started by graduates of either Maternity Center Association or the Frontier School of Midwifery and Family Nursing. Curriculum was quickly standardized and shared, making the establishment of new nurse-midwifery programs relatively easy. As of the fall of 2000, there were 5 post-secondary educational programs and 40 graduate programs in nurse-midwifery, with one direct entry midwifery program accredited or pre-accredited by the American College of Nurse-Midwives (ACNM) Division of Accreditation (DOA) (ACNM, DOA, 2000).

The Professional Association

Of particular historical importance in the development of nurse-midwifery in the U.S. was the establishment of the American College of Nurse-Midwifery (ACNM) in 1955 (which became the American College of Nurse-Midwives in 1969), a professional association distinct from both medicine and nursing though collaborating with both on issues of mutual concern (Varney, 1997). ACNM defines the nurse-midwife as educated in the two disciplines of nursing and midwifery, and autonomous in providing midwifery care for healthy childbearing women and their newborns, while working within a health care system as team members with physicians and nurses. This commitment to collaboration with physicians and nurses on behalf of seamless care for women and their families has affected the organization and content of the educational programs since 1932, with many physician and nurse colleagues providing specialized content as guest lecturers and consultants.

As Burst (1991) noted, the development and strengthening of the American College of Nurse-Midwives has made all the difference in the education and practice of nurse-midwifery today. In 1957, the ACNM Committee on Curriculum and Accreditation was formed, and in 1962, the National League for Nursing decided it could not accredit nurse-midwifery programs because not all of them were in graduate schools of nursing. This meant that the ACNM would have to develop its own accrediting mechanism and define what should be included in educational programs. The first nurse-midwifery programs to be accredited by a voluntary process were in 1968. In 1974, the Committee name changed to the Division of Approval, and today it is known as the ACNM Division of Accreditation (DOA), and received recognition by the U.S. Department of Education in 1984 as an accrediting agency for nurse-midwifery. "The DOA sought this recognition as testimony to the quality of our process" (Conway-Welch, 1986, p. 13). Of great importance to setting the criteria for the accreditation of nurse-midwifery educational programs was the delineation of the essential knowledge, skills, and behaviors needed for the practice of midwifery. The ACNM Education Committee formally defined the "core competencies" in nurse-midwifery that strengthened the definition of content (both theory and clinical) to be included in any nurse-midwifery educational program—whether at the certificate, master's, or doctoral level. These core competencies have been revised and updated periodically to reflect the expanding scope of midwifery practice from childbearing care to include family planning and well women (gynecological) health care (all current ACNM accreditation documents can be obtained from the ACNM).

The ACNM's development of a national certification examination in the late 1960s, with formal adoption on May 1, 1971, also served to assure the public of the safety and competence of any graduate in nurse-midwifery as s/he enter into practice (Foster, 1986). The fact that many states then included this national certification as a requirement for licensure of the nurse-midwife strengthened the public's support and acceptance of nurse-midwifery care. A Task Analysis of nurse-midwifery practice is completed every 5 years to determine that the national examination now offered by the ACNM Certification Council, Inc. (ACC) reflects current practice (Fullerton, 1994).

In summary, the key influences of having a strong professional association for nurse-midwives and midwifery practice include 1) setting and standardizing the criteria for the education of nurse-midwives, 2) establishing a national certification examination for entry into practice, 3) setting and monitoring the standards of midwifery practice through peer review, 4) defining the philosophy of midwifery care and a code of ethics for its practitioners, and 5) working for and achieving legal recognition for the practice of nurse-midwifery in every state and territory in the U.S.

Summary of the Development of Nurse-Midwifery

Nurse-midwifery in the United States developed slowly but with ever-increasing strength from 1925 to the early 1970s. It had the benefit of wonderful traditions of safe and satisfying care provided by the often well-trained immigrant midwives and the granny midwives in the South. While struggles to attain respect and recognition were at times difficult, the fact that nurse-midwifery merged the two disciplines of midwifery and nursing helped give status to the nurse-midwife and access to the variety of established health care systems not available to the indigenous midwives in the early 1900s. Support from well-respected obstetricians also helped the development of nurse-midwifery. Of special note was the formal recognition of the practice of nurse-midwifery in 1972 with the adoption of a joint statement by the American College of Obstetricians and Gynecologists (ACOG) and the ACNM. Strong, standardized educational programs, national certification for entry into practice, licensure to practice in accord with standards, and a strong professional organization have provided the solid foundation for the current practice of midwifery in the U.S.

HISTORY OF THE NURSE PRACTITIONER MOVEMENT

During the 1960s activists called for a reform of the health care system. Medical specialization, which had increased dramatically after World War II, had decreased the availability of physicians to provide general medical care. In addition, the distribution of the supply of physicians was uneven, leaving many areas in the country underserved. Coupled with this shortage of family and general practice physicians was an increasing belief that nurses should expand their scope of practice, particularly in the area of ambulatory care.

A number of nursing care demonstrations were carried out in the late 1960s. The first of these that was reported was at the University of Colorado where Loretta Ford, a nurse, and Henry Silver, a physician, developed a program to prepare pediatric nurses to provide primary health care services to children. They believed that specially trained nurses could bridge the gap between the health care needs of children and the availability of pediatric primary care services. Nurses were expected to provide comprehensive well care services, manage minor acute illness, and manage stable chronic illness in children. These nurses were trained to provide services in clinics or physicians' offices in areas without adequate access to primary health care (Ford & Silver, 1967).

Surprisingly, the American Medical Association's Committee on Nursing in 1970 supported the concept of the nurse practitioner. We can with hindsight speculate that physicians anticipated that even though the nurse's role was expanding it would not alter the physician-nurse relationship and certainly would not create competition with physicians.

Some nursing leaders were supportive of the new role, while others felt that nurse practitioners had abandoned nursing and were practicing medicine (Rogers, 1972). In 1971 federal support for expanding the role of nurses was assured with a report to the Secretary of Health, Education and Welfare titled *Extending the Scope of Nursing Practice* (The Secretary's Committee to Study Extended Roles for Nurses, 1971). This report called for nurses to expand their roles, collect medical information and make clinical decisions about patient care. Expanding the role of nurses was seen as the solution to the problem of inadequate access to health services.

The federal government funded many of the original programs preparing nurse practitioners (NPs). The majority of these programs were codirected by nurses and physicians and were located in continuing education departments or regional medical program offices. There was no standard for entry into NP practice. Individuals with diplomas, associate degrees, bachelor's degrees and master's degrees were all accepted into these certificate-granting programs. The NP concept, although continuously controversial, expanded significantly in the late 1960s and in the 1970s. Numerous programs, some quickly formed and of variable quality, were developed. By 1977, 117 certificate programs and 61 master's programs were in place (Sultz, Zielezny, Gentry, & Kinyon, 1978). By the 1980s the trend toward certificate programs slowed and the number of master's programs expanded. By then NPs were prepared to deliver primary care to children, adults, and families.

In 1973, the Division of Nursing of the United States Public Health Service funded a major study of NP practice. The results of the study were favorable to the NP role and the study became the basis for continued funding of programs to prepare NPs (Sultz et al., 1978). Studies performed since then have continually been favorable to NP practice. Most studies compare the work of NPs with the work of physicians even though NPs would argue that their approach in primary care is based on health whereas a physician's approach is based on disease. In 1986, a report by the Office of Technology Assessment (OTA) found NPs' practice to be equal to physician's practice. However, they found that NPs scored higher on quality of care items than their physician colleagues and focused more on health promotion activities (OTA, 1986).

By the 1980s NP practice was well established, particularly in areas where reimbursement was not an issue, such as Health Maintenance Organizations and publicly funded ambulatory care settings. The number of NPs had grown from approximately 250 in 1970 to 20,000 by 1980 (Sultz, Henry, Kinyon, Buck, &

Bullough, 1983). Today NPs practice in a variety of sites: acute care hospitals, emergency rooms, family practice settings, nursing homes, neonatal intensive care units, occupational health offices, oncology settings, community clinics, physician's offices, mental hospitals, schools, colleges, prisons. Between 1992 and 1997, the number of master's level NP programs increased from fewer than 100 to more than 250. Enrollment in programs increased dramatically. The result has been an increase in the number of graduating NPs from 1,500 in 1992 to 6,350 in 1997, and expected to continue to increase. The estimated number of practicing NPs in 1997 was 63,000 (Cooper, Laud, & Dietrich, 1998).

RECURRING THEMES AND LESSONS FOR MIDWIFERY AND ADVANCED PRACTICE NURSING

As one reviews the brief history of midwifery, nurse-midwifery, and the nurse practitioner movement presented in this chapter, it is interesting to note several important similarities as well as the few differences between the development of midwifery and the development of nurse practitioners. The similarities include 1) the willingness of both groups of nurses to care for the vulnerable, the rural, and the poor—especially in those areas where physicians choose not to practice; 2) the rise in use due to shortages of physicians; 3) the belief that nurses should and could expand their scope of practice into primary care; 4) an early belief that competition between nurses/midwives and physicians would not materialize; 5) the importance of the support of influential physicians; 6) an ongoing uncertainty and struggle with organized medicine to allow both nurse-midwives and nurse practitioners to practice in an autonomous manner; 7) significant support by key governmental agencies, including financial support from the Division of Nursing, Health and Human Services; 8) a commitment to university-based education; and 9) recognition of the political voice needed to promote these advanced practice nurses and midwives as viable health professionals who make a significant contribution to the health of this nation, especially its most vulnerable citizens.

One of the major differences in the historical development of nurse-midwives and nurse practitioners relates to the longer traditions of midwifery and the strength of the American College of Nurse-Midwives with its definition and standardization of educational criteria, standards of practice, and scope of practice. The nurse practitioners have a much less defined (and wider) scope of practice, less agreement on basic competencies until recent years, and no specialty accreditation of the educational programs, even though they are more numerous than nurse-midwives. It is these similarities and differences that inform current curricula in nurse-midwifery/midwifery and nurse practitioner education.

SUMMARY

The practice of midwifery by nurse-midwives and direct entry midwives has a long tradition of excellence, with safety being the defining characteristic, along with meeting the needs of patients and valuing the collaboration with physician and nurse colleagues. Decades of evidence support the cost-quality effectiveness of both midwifery care and the care given by nurse practitioners. Public acceptance of both roles is on the increase, though the battle to maintain autonomy of practice continues. That battle can only be won with excellent care, political savvy, and patient support. Preparing clinicians of the future requires that teachers focus on the competencies needed for safe, satisfying, high quality care. The new teacher would be wise to read and understand the history and development of both disciplines to understand how and why the educational curricula and expectations of graduates have evolved. This understanding and the lessons learned from history can support and define how we are to proceed in the future, ever mindful of the need to focus on what our patients need and how we can work together to meet those needs.

REFERENCES

American College of Nurse-Midwives, Division of Accreditation. (2000). *List of ACNM pre-accredited and accredited educational programs.* Washington, DC: ACNM.

American Nurses Association. (1993). *A meta-analysis of process of care, clinical outcomes, and cost effectiveness of nurses in primary care roles: Nurse practitioners and nurse-midwives.* [Executive Summary]. Washington, DC: Author.

Breckinridge, M. (1952). *Wide neighborhoods: A story of the frontier nursing service.* Lexington, KY: University of Kentucky Press.

Burst, H. V. (1991). The American College of Nurse-Midwives: Representing an ancient profession reborn in contemporary society. *Midwife means with woman.* [Video]. Bethesda, MD: National Library of Medicine.

CMI. Medical Mission Sisters (1994). *50th Celebration reunion: Remembering CMI/Santa Fe.* Video available from MMS U.S. Headquarters, 8400 Pine Road, Philadelphia, PA.

Conway-Welch, C. (1986). Assuring the quality of nurse-midwifery education: The ACNM Division of Accreditation. In J. Rooks & J. E. Haas (Eds.), *Nurse-midwifery in America* (pp. 10–13). Washington, DC: ACNM.

Cooper, R. A., Laud, P., & Dietrich, C. L. (1998). Current and projected workforce of nonphysician clinicians. *Journal of the American Medical Association, 280*(9), 788–794.

Ford, L. C., & Silver, H. K. (1967). Expanded role of the nurse in child care. *Nursing Outlook, 15,* 43–45.

Foster, J. C. (1986). Ensuring competence of nurse-midwives at entrance into the profession: The national certification examination. In J. Rooks & J. E. Haas (Eds.), *Nurse-midwifery in America* (pp. 14–16). Washington, DC: ACNM.

Fullerton, J. T. (1994). A task analysis of American certified nurse-midwifery. *Journal of Nurse-Midwifery, 39,* 348–357.

Hegel, G. W. F. (1832). *Werke.* Germany: Duncker.

Levy, B. S., Wilkinson, F. S., & Marine, W. M. (1971). Reducing neonatal mortality rate with nurse-midwives. *American Journal of Obstetrics and Gynecology, 109,* 50–58.

Litoff, J. B. (1978). *American midwives: 1860 to the present.* Westport, CT: Greenwood Press.

Lynaugh, J. (1991). *Introduction to National Library of Medicine symposium on midwifery.* [Video]. Bethesda, MD: National Library of Medicine.

Maternity Center Association. (1955). *Twenty years of nurse-midwifery: 1933–1953.* New York: Author.

Metropolitan Life Insurance Company. (1958). Summary of the tenth thousand confinement records of the Frontier Nursing Service. *FNS Quarterly Bulletin, 33*(4), 44–55.

Office of Technology Assessment. (1986). Nurse practitioners, physician assistants, and certified nurse-midwives: A policy analysis. *Health Technology Case Study, 37.* Washington, DC: U.S. Government Printing Office.

Record, J., & Cohen, H. (1972). The introduction of midwifery in a prepaid group practice. *American Journal of Public Health, 62,* 354–360.

Robinson, S. (1984). A historical development of midwifery in the black community: 1600–1940. *Journal of Nurse-Midwifery, 29*(4), 247–250.

Rogers, M. E. (1972). Nursing: To be or not to be? *Nursing Outlook, 20,* 42–48.

Rooks, J. P. (1997). *Midwifery and childbirth in America.* Philadelphia: Temple University Press.

Rooks, J. P., Weatherby, N. L., Ernst, E. K. M., Stapleton, S., Rosen, D., & Rosenfield, A. (1989). Outcomes of care in birth centers: The National Birth Center Study. *New England Journal of Medicine, 321,* 1804–1811.

Shoemaker, Sister M. (1947). *History of nurse-midwifery in the United States.* Washington, DC: Catholic University of America Press.

Sultz, H. A., Zielezny, M., Gentry, J. M., & Kinyon, L. (1978). *Longitudinal Study of Nurse Practitioners, Phase II* (DHEW publication No. HRA 78-92). Washington, DC: U.S. Government Printing Office.

Sultz, H. A., Henry, O. M., Kinyon, L. J., Buck, G. M., & Bullough, B. (1983). A decade of change for nurse practitioners: Program Highlights 1. *Nursing Outlook, 31,* 131–141, 188.

The Secretary's Committee to Study Extended Roles for Nurses. (1971). *Extending the scope of nursing practice.* Washington, DC: U.S. Government Printing Office.

Thompson, J. (1981). Nurse-midwives and health promotion during pregnancy. In R. Lederman, B. Raff, & P. Carroll (Eds.), *Perinatal parental behavior: Nursing research and implications for newborn health* (pp. 29–57). New York: Liss.

Thompson, J. E. (1986). Nurse-midwifery care: 1925 to 1984. In H. Werley, J. Fitzpatrick, & R. L. Taunton (Eds.), *Annual review of nursing research* (Vol. 4, pp. 153–173). New York: Springer Publishing.

Thompson, J. B. (1986). Safety and effectiveness of nurse-midwifery care: Research review. In J. Rooks & J. E. Haas (Eds.), *Nurse-midwifery in America* (pp. 40–44). Washington, DC: American College of Nurse-Midwives.

Thompson, J. E., Oakley, D., Burke, M., Jay, S., & Conklin, M. (1989). Theory building in nurse-midwifery: The care process. *Journal of Nurse-Midwifery, 34*(3), 120–130.

Thompson, J. E., Walsh, L. V., & Merkatz, I. R. (1990). The history of prenatal care: Cultural, social and medical contexts. In I. R. Merkatz & J. E. Thompson (Eds.), *New perspectives on prenatal care* (pp. 9–30). New York: Elsevier.

Ulrich, L. T. (1990). *A midwife's tale: The life of Martha Ballard based on her diary, 1785–1812.* New York: Alfred A. Knopf.

Varney, H. (1997). *Varney's midwifery* (3rd ed.). Boston: Jones and Bartlett Publishers.

Walsh, L. V. (1991). *Midwife means with woman: An historical perspective.* [Brochure to accompany National Library of Medicine video]. Washington, DC: ACNM.

Wertz, R. W., & Wertz, D. C. (1977). *Lying in: A history of childbirth in America.* New York: The Free Press.

CHAPTER 2

Making the Transition From Clinician to Teacher

It is not only the change from one role to another; it is the whole range of human experience—one's own and that of others—that constitutes the dynamics of the transition.

—J. E. Mulligan, "Professional Transition: Nurse to Nurse-Midwife"

SUGGESTED OUTCOMES FOR THIS CHAPTER

At the end of this chapter, the reader will be able to

1. understand the major elements of transition theory in nursing,
2. describe the indicators of successful role transition applied to teaching, and
3. describe the content and use of transitions seminars in teacher preparation.

INTRODUCTION

There are many transitions in our lives. From child to adult, from nurse to nurse practitioner or nurse-midwife, and from clinician to teacher are but a few of those that come to mind. A transition as defined by Chick and Meleis (1986) is a "passage from one life phase, condition or status to another" (p. 239). Meleis has spent many years exploring and understanding the transitions that nurses go through during their professional careers. The focus of this chapter is to describe some of the transitions that expert clinicians go through as they take on the role of teacher in advanced practice nursing and midwifery programs (Esper, 1995). In addition, the use of transitions seminars to facilitate the move from clinician to teacher will be described, based on the creative work of Jerrilyn Hobdy and Vivian Lowenstein. These nurse-midwifery educators pioneered the development and use of such seminars at the University of Pennsylvania School of Nursing's program in nurse-midwifery to support the transition of learners from nurse to nurse-midwife.

ELEMENTS OF TRANSITIONS THEORY IN NURSING

Schumacher and Meleis (1994) summarized the review of transitions theory as used in nursing and by a variety of authors in three categories: 1) the types of transitions addressed in the literature, 2) conditions that influence transitions, and 3) indicators of healthy transitions. They noted several universal or common properties of transitions in nursing. The first transition of importance to novice teachers is the recognition that the process of transition takes time—it is not accomplished at a moment's notice or just because we wish it to happen. Allowing oneself to learn the new role, understanding that a certain level of discomfort is normal until one can gain the confidence of an advanced beginner, and holding on to the understanding that wisdom and confidence come with experience help to explain the time needed to make a successful transition from expert clinician to teacher.

During the time that one is in transition, there are phases or stages of moving from one role to another, and one can visualize movement toward the new, desired role. A second commonality in the transition from expert clinician to novice teacher is that a variety of changes will occur in the individual. These changes occur in one's view of oneself (identity), in the roles and relationships one is developing, and in one's pattern of behavior. For example, an expert clinician may have an initial view of themselves as less than competent in the new teaching role. This can be an uncomfortable feeling, yet common when anyone goes from the familiar to the unfamiliar. Patience with oneself during this time is important. New teachers are also encouraged to allow themselves time to learn their new role just as they will allow their advanced practice nurse or midwifery learners time to learn the clinical role they have chosen. Another example relates to changes in behavior. The behavior of the clinician as a primary caregiver will give way to the behavior of a teacher in situations where the APN or midwifery learner is the primary caregiver and the teacher more of an observer in the situation. It took one of the authors over a year to accept the challenge and role of midwifing the student rather than the client, and to experience a similar level of joy and satisfaction in this type of role.

As one proceeds on the path of discovery and begins to understand key transition points, the authors believe it is helpful for the new teacher to keep in mind some of the systems involved in this transition, conditions that may influence the quality of this transition, and the markers that one can use to tell when a transition point or stage has been accomplished or successful. The systems involved in transition include changes in identity, roles, relationships, abilities, and patterns of behavior, as described below.

Types of Transitions

Chick and Meleis (1986) identified three types of transitions that nurses face during their nursing activities. These included developmental, situational, and health-illness transitions. Schumacher and Meleis (1994) added a fourth type of transition in their review of the nursing literature—that of organizational transition. Each will be explored briefly in relation to the growth and development of a clinician-teacher.

Developmental transition relates to significant life events of particular importance to women, such as pregnancy, parenthood, adolescence, midlife, and menopause. Since nursing and midwifery are primarily female professions, these developmental transitions are very relevant. The take-home point for the developing teacher is that the transition from clinician to teacher involves the whole person—and that person needs to be aware of any developmental life events that are going on simultaneously with the role change to teacher. Imagine yourself adjusting to parenthood as you are also adjusting to being a novice teacher. This is just one possible scenario for the new teacher, and reflects the complex and intricate interaction and balance of competing priorities that characterize many transitions in life.

Situational transitions are those that arise when we change our educational and professional roles. Situational transitions are those of most importance in this text, as the nurse practitioner or midwife clinicians begin both the educational transition to learning about teaching, as well as the role transition to teacher. The authors were unable to find specific literature support for this important transition from expert clinician to teacher in a clinical discipline such as nursing. However, the extrapolation of transitions theory applied to nursing and other events in one's life is natural. These transitions often require a change in the environment of learning and practice from a clinical setting to an academic setting. The transitions also include a dramatic change in functions and scope of practice (Reed-McKay, 1989), as the teacher learns to carry major responsibility for helping others learn while also learning their new role.

The health-illness transitions found in the nursing literature often refer to the effects of specific illness conditions (acute or chronic) on the lives of those affected, including patients and significant others around them. Brooten and colleagues (1988) addressed the transition from hospital to home for very low birthweight infants and their families, just one example of a major transition in levels of health and illness care for individuals. Though the transition from clinical practice to teaching does not directly involve a change in one's health status, if one is not in the best of health during this transition many of the required changes will be more difficult.

Organizational transitions refer to transitions in the environment of organizations. One of the more prominent examples of an organizational change that can affect the development of new teachers is a change in leadership within the academic setting. Changing one's primary mentor, changing one's teacher colleagues early in the transition process, or living through the potential upset of a change in the director or dean of the academic unit can precipitate emotional, physical, as well as psychological sequelae in the developing teacher. These responses, whether positive or negative, must be acknowledged and understood so that they do not adversely affect the teacher's performance in the classroom or practice setting. One cannot ignore the organization or environment of teaching and learning, and must be knowledgeable of the expectations required (see chapter 14).

Factors That Influence Transitions

As noted above, there are several factors that influence both the process of transition from clinician to teacher and the time it takes to comfortably accept the new role and functions. The conditions that influence the quality of transition from clinician to teacher include meanings, expectations, level of knowledge and skill, environment, level of planning, and emotional and physical well-being (adapted from Meleis et al., 2000; Schumacher & Meleis, 1994). Meaning is one's appraisal of what is to be expected in changing from clinician to teacher, and what one anticipates as the major effects this change will have on their lives. This meaning may be either positive or negative, and must be understood from the perspective of those who are experiencing it (Adlersberg & Thorne, 1990). The use of transitions seminars discussed later in this chapter assist the new teacher in reflecting on their projected role as teacher, what they think or anticipate will happen in to them in this role, and why they are learning to be a teacher. Sharing such personal insight through guided imagery or other techniques can assist the learner in moving along the phases of transition with understanding and knowing.

Expectations of the role of teacher in the clinical discipline also affect the transition process. How many times has the clinician worked with patients who had unrealistic expectations of how they would respond to a pregnancy or a new diagnosis of asthma or diabetes? Consider the effort, knowledge, and support needed to help these patients come to a more realistic understanding of what that condition means and will demand of the individual. This very same effort is needed in helping the new teacher come to grips with the realistic demands of teaching along with the excitement and enthusiasm for carrying out this important role. This is where the importance of selecting and working with a mentor teacher is evident.

Transition from clinician to teacher also requires a level of knowledge and skill that may not be readily apparent at the beginning of this journey. Since many of us have been exposed to teachers who assumed that just because they were expert clinicians who worked well with patients, they could automatically be good teachers as well. It is true that expert clinicians are good patient teachers, but this does not automatically translate into working with adult learners who are eager to learn the very role that the expert clinician excels in. Adding the classroom and asynchronous learning environment does influence teacher effectiveness, and adding the APN or midwifery learner into the patient care equation also changes the teaching/learning environment as noted later on in this text. Suffice it to say, there is a great deal of learning and knowledge, and many skills and behaviors needed to become a successful teacher in advanced practice nursing and midwifery. Understanding this fact and setting one's course on learning all that is needed to proceed will facilitate the transition from clinician to teacher of clinicians.

The environment of learning to be a teacher can either facilitate or detract from the transition process (MacNeil, 1997). As noted earlier, the selection and use of a mentor teacher and observations of a variety of role models in teaching are helpful resources during this professional transition. As noted by Grady (1992), Rice (1988), and Wuest (1990), an experienced teacher serving as a role model and mentor can pave the transition road by being a guide and a sounding board for discussion of transition points along the way and strategies to address the next phase of transition. The sociocultural context of transition from clinician to teacher is similar in part to the transition from nurse to nurse-midwife or advanced practice nurse in that there can be a gap between the social status and culture of the teacher and the learner. Culture often directs how an individual responds to learning a new role, the support network that will be developed, and the trust levels expected. If the move from clinician to teacher involves a reduction in salary, socioeconomic factors can potentially influence the smoothness of the transition.

Planning for transition from clinician to teacher is an important process. If the new teacher can identify the problems, issues, needs, and reasons for moving from clinician to teacher, the transition process often proceeds more smoothly. One of the important considerations in any transition is that a wide range of emotions will be experienced, whether one has long cherished the new role or been recruited into it with much initial resistance. Several emotions have been identified in the nursing literature related to transitions in one's career. These include anxiety, insecurity, frustration, depression, apprehension, ambivalence, role conflict and low self-esteem, fear of failure, and unwarranted self-criticism (Schumacher & Meleis, 1994). It is noteworthy that there is no mention of more positive emotions like joy, anticipation, and excitement that the authors of this text felt in their transitions from clinicians to teachers. This is one area where a positive mentor teacher, while acknowledging that there will be moments of anxiety and fear of the unknown, can promote the enthusiasm and excitement for what the teacher role can be and is. The support and understanding of mentor teachers is vital in the progression of the new teacher transition.

Characteristics of Successful Transitions

Signs that the transition from clinician to teacher of clinicians is progressing normally and in a healthy manner include a sense of personal well-being that is accompanied by mastery of new behaviors (successful learning leads to a willingness to take on even more complex learning with both the risks and benefits accepted), and a confidence in the goodness of fit of new relationships. The initial feelings of anxiety and fear of the unknown are replaced with confidence, dignity, and a general sense of a quality life. A feeling of competence in teaching based on knowledge and skills learned, practiced, and repeated, replaces the earlier feelings of inadequacy that novice teachers often express. One of the greatest challenges of the mentor teacher is to constantly remind the novice teacher that they bring many important competencies to the teaching role—they are not starting from ground zero. One of the authors of this text encouraged new learners to post signs in their living quarters that reminded them of their life experience and competencies on a daily basis, such as "I am a very competent nurse-midwife" or "I know how to teach others" or "I am an eager learner and successful in learning." Hollander and Haber (1992) note that intervention during transition is important, and should be directed at diminishing the disruptive aspects of new relationships and promoting the development of new relationships. The authors' use of transitions seminars during their teacher education program includes support for the development of new teacher relationships among the learners in this program, providing support and reinforcement of the normality of what is happening to them during this transition.

Application of transitions theory to the major role change of clinician to teacher of clinicians is, in some ways, traveling into uncharted territory. The authors continue their journey to stretch the boundaries of transitions theory and invite the reader to join them as we all discover more about ourselves as teachers and learners. Teaching in advanced practice nursing and midwifery is exciting, fun, rewarding, and makes a difference in the lives of our patients. Successful passage through the transition of role change and growth of self are the expected outcomes. The remainder of this chapter will describe the major teaching method the authors have found useful in promoting healthy and successful transition from expert clinician to teacher of the next generation of advanced practice nurses and midwives.

TRANSITION SEMINARS: ROLE CHANGE AND SUPPORT

The successful transition from expert clinician to teacher requires support, guidance, and direction in the early phases of change. The teaching method used (with positive feedback from teacher-learners) has been specially designed transitions seminars offered at set points in the Teacher Education Program (TEP) run by the authors. This program is a nontraditional post-master's certificate program that includes 3 full weeks of seminars and microteaching on the campus of the University of Pennsylvania with each week separated by 3 months of planned activities with a mentor teacher at the home university. The transitions seminars are used as the beginning and end of each of the 1 week sessions on the Penn campus. The series of seminars are designed to help learners with the process of changing to a new role.

Too often, the focus of APN and midwifery education is primarily on the cognitive and psychomotor domains of learning, with limited attention to the affective domain. The transitions seminars focus on the affective aspects of learning. The affective domain identifies the feelings, belief systems, and values of individuals in relation to life choices and events that result from those choices. The reader is encouraged to think of creative ways to plan and use transitions seminars in their own setting and in their own transition to the teaching role. The description of the TEP transitions seminars are offered as one example.

Transitions seminars are flexible and have been used for different groups of learners, i.e. nurses, nurse-midwives, nurse practitioners, and teachers, to support and facilitate the process of change. The seminars are semi-structured and focus upon the individual and group processes. Master teachers are the best facilitators of the transition from clinician to teacher for they have years of observation and experience with how that transition occurs. Master teachers are often in the best position to observe the behaviors of new teachers (learners), which may exhibit the struggles and lack of confidence that learners feel. When new teachers are given the opportunity to express their feelings about this process, they have a better understanding of who they are as individuals and as a group, and how to be successful in achieving their new role.

As master teachers, the authors have observed patterns of new teacher "ups and downs" throughout the 9-month teacher education program at the University of Pennsylvania School of Nursing. By being alert to such patterns, the master teacher can intervene in a timely manner to address the problems individually or within the group. The authors have learned over time that group support and discussion of the highs and lows of learning to teach can be very important and reassuring—allowing all members of the group to hear that they are not alone in their crisis of confidence, their sense of loss of control, or their less than perfect class day, as well as rejoicing in their times of great success and positive feedback from those they are teaching.

The Role of the Faculty

What is different about transitions seminars is that the faculty takes a "back seat"—asking open-ended questions, planning small group activities—and listening—allowing the developing teachers time to experience how they feel and to learn from one another. The faculty's emphasis on listening reflects their belief that this is the learner's time to gain a perspective of what is happening to them. It is strongly suggested that master teachers provide for continuity of support to the group. Prior to each seminar the faculty review the objectives for the seminar and also discuss the role each will take for different parts of the seminar. For example, one will take the role as the facilitator for a discussion while the other observes the group process. One faculty member will do the readings at the beginning of the seminar and another might do the readings for the end. The faculty works as a "seamless" team, supporting one another, having an understanding of how they together would create the learning environment, while also being accepting of each other's differences (strengths). The faculty also meet at the end of the seminar to evaluate the group process and any changes in the content, process, or role of the faculty for the next time the seminar is offered.

The Objectives of the Transitions Seminars in the TEP Program

The authors established the following objectives for the transitions seminars used in the Teacher Education Program.

At the completion of these transitions seminars, the learner will be able to

1. demonstrate an awareness of communication that facilitates caring for one's own and others' needs in the development of the teacher role;
2. identify your preferred learning style and how you would like to expand your abilities to work with a variety of learners;
3. identify and describe the process of change as it applies to one's identity, roles, relationships, abilities, and patterns of behavior;

4. record key "transition points" on the journey from master clinician to novice teacher; and

5. clearly define the role of novice teacher and describe your desired goals as a teacher.

Transitions Guidelines (The Rules of the Game)

At the beginning of the first seminar, the faculty should review the purpose and goals of the seminars and the guidelines for the group. The guidelines help to set the tone and the environment, which should be supportive, respectful, and positive. (These can be developed by the faculty and the learners.) The following guidelines were developed and worked well for the TEP seminars, based on the work of Lowenstein and Hobdy.

1. There are no required books, no syllabus, or exams for these seminars. (A sense of humor, however, is required!) All learners are asked to put away any books or papers, clear the space in front of them, and thus set the tone for clearing the mind of outside demands in order to concentrate or focus on the task at hand—that of thinking about what it means to be a teacher and what is happening to oneself.

2. Confidentiality of what occurs in the discussions should be respected. (What is said in the room should not go outside.)

3. Everyone is allowed to be right. Respect that everyone has a right to their perspective of how they see the world.

4. The seminars are not meant for psychological therapy. They are meant to support and facilitate the process of role transition.

5. Individuals may choose not to share in discussions or participate in activities.

6. Each seminar follows the same format: readings and a minute of silence at the beginning and end of the seminar, discussions/activities in the middle.

7. It is expected that everyone will be present for the seminar, though not required to talk or share personal insights until comfortable doing so.

8. Written evaluations are requested at the end of each week, including an evaluation of the transitions time and suggestions for future seminars.

THE SEMINARS

The seminars should be planned as a series. In general, the number of seminars depends upon the length of the program, the times when learners are on campus, are facing new challenges, or at the request of the learners. There were times when learners would tell the faculty that they felt the need to have time to discuss issues that affected their professional role in a transitions seminar that had not been planned. The new teachers are also encouraged to plan for their own transitions seminars at their home university during the 3 months of home activity in learning the teaching role.

The seminars should be scheduled at times when learners have less anxiety (not the day of an exam or before a paper is due), and they have time to process how they're feeling (without worrying about the next class, their microteaching assignment, etc.). The scheduling of the TEP transitions seminars reflected the fact that participants often traveled great distances to get to the program, had to rearrange their entire life to have the week at Penn, and were juggling a variety of responsibilities as well as learning to be a teacher. The TEP transitions seminars began each week's program and were the last event at the end of each week. (See sample questions that follow.)

Each seminar has the same structure. A reading is done at the beginning and end of the seminar to help individuals center on themselves. The TEP faculty added relaxing or meditation music to the background of the readings and period of silence that has added a calming effect to the environment. Then there is a moment of silence to continue the process of centering and to "be here now." A discussion/activity is planned for the main portion of the seminar which focuses on the purpose of that seminar. Two or three different discussions/activities enable individuals to experience their role transition in different ways.

The first seminar begins to foster communication, sharing of oneself and the building of the group. After the reading(s) and the minute of silence, the learners may be asked to find a person that they do not know in the group. For approximately 5 minutes they should give the other person information about themselves related to how they would like to be introduced. The group then comes together and each pair introduces each other to the group. The participants learn of each other's lifestyles, experiences, hobbies, and goals. The second part of the seminar often is a group building exercise/game which fosters trust, the art of negotiation, and competition, while helping individuals to identify what roles they take in different circumstances (e.g., leadership, active/passive).

The end of the week seminar focuses on role transitions and what has happened during the week. Following the readings and silence, questions are asked toward identifying what role the learner is in now and how that feels. The next part of the seminar questions how the learner plans to use what they have learned during this week at their home university. Some seminars will also include role-playing or trigger films of simulated experiences that will trigger discussion of the various aspects of role transition for the new teacher. These simulations should identify ethical/challenging decision-making for new teachers as individuals and as a group. Another exercise is identifying how each individual learns, a discussion of how that affects one's role (as a teacher and a learner), and the ability to apply the information to different teaching and learning experiences in the educational program (theoretical and clinical learning experiences).

Transitions seminar content that new teachers can use with their own students might focus on the chosen profession of the group (nursing, advanced practice, midwifery). The history and documents of the profession/educational institution (philosophy, mission statement, code of ethics) are discussed. This gives an opportunity for students to identify their values, beliefs, and how they fit into their new chosen role. Inviting individuals who are role models to the seminar to discuss their transitional experiences with students is helpful. An inspirational film/video or reading about the profession can be used for the second part of the seminar.

During the second and third weeks of the TEP, the transitions seminars focus on various phases and transition points in the lives of the developing teacher. The last transitions seminar provides some closure to the group experience and recognition of the new role of teacher. The discussion begins with remembering the first transition seminar—where one began—and then examining where one is now. The focus is on what occurred along the way, the positive experiences, the supportive people, the individuals' strengths, and the feelings that accompanied transitions. Individuals are given the opportunity to discuss their plans of how to continue the process of growth and supportive environments (E-mail surely helps, and the listserve developed for each class of TEP graduates is maintained for such communication). Open-ended statements are used for the last part of the seminar, encouraging individuals to focus on the future: "The hardest thing ahead of me is . . . " and then, "The thing I most look forward to is. . . . " The seminar ends with a reading that offers a positive, uplifting sense for the group.

Selection of Transition Readings

One of the fun parts of teaching is looking for inspirational writings about what we love to do. The choices of readings for transitions seminars reflect the joy, work, enthusiasm, challenge, and rewards of teaching in advanced practice nursing and midwifery. These choices are personal, and will reflect the individual teacher's beliefs about teaching and learning, their identification of what is needed by the group to facilitate their transition, and what is meaningful to the teacher, for teachers of teachers require attention to their own needs for transition and learning. Individual participants also are encouraged to bring readings to the seminars, from inspirational leaders, poets, historians, and contemporary writers. Whatever the selection, the authors encourage the leaders of transitions seminars to make sure they fit with the purpose of the seminar at that time.

Selected Questions for Teacher Education Transitions Seminars

Activities and Questions for Seminar I—Beginning of Program

1. Think about why you decided to come to the TEP program.
2. In thinking about the journey into teaching that you are beginning, what are you looking forward to? Complete the following sentence, "The hardest thing ahead of me is . . . "
3. What are the gifts/talents that you bring to this new role? What do you anticipate as your most important needs for change (identity, relationships, abilities, patterns of behavior) along this road to teaching?
4. Complete the following statements:
   The best teacher I ever had was . . . because . . .
   The worst teacher I ever had was . . . because . . .
5. How do you learn best? (Learning Style Inventory completed and discussed.)

End of First Week Seminar

1. What has happened to you during this week?
2. How will what you have learned affect your teaching?
3. How will you convey your role change to others?
4. What are you looking forward to in the next 3 months?

Beginning of Second Week Seminar

1. What has happened to you during the past few months in your home university? Where are you now? What changes have occurred in your teaching role?
2. What barriers/limitations did you overcome in this new role (personal, professional, system, time, etc.)?
3. What transition points did you identify?
4. What successes in teaching did you experience and why?
5. What areas of your teaching role are you currently working on?
6. What are you looking forward to during this week? What is your goal for the week?
7. How can we facilitate your growth in teaching this week?

End of Second Week Seminar

1. What has happened to you during this week? What are the significant things you learned about yourself this week?

2. What has been your response to thinking about teaching in the clinical setting? What new clinical teaching strategies will you try out?
3. How will what you have learned this week affect your teaching in the next few months? What are the major challenges facing you in the next 3 months of teaching? How will you deal with them?
4. How will you convey your role changes to others?
5. What are you looking forward to in the next 3 months?

Beginning of Third Week Seminar

1. We have come to the last session in this teacher education program. What are the thoughts that come into your mind as you prepare for this last week together?
2. What are the major transition points you have noticed during these past 9 months? How have you responded to them?
3. Please share any new insight into clinical teaching that you gained during the past 3 months.
4. What is your goal for this week of learning together?

Final Transitions Seminar

1. What are the thoughts that come to mind as you prepare to say goodbye to the participants in this teacher education program?
2. What are the strengths and limitations of using planned "transitions" seminars in your own teaching?
3. What are the professional teaching goals you have set for yourself in the coming year?

Each of these seminars began and ended with silence and selected readings.

Recognizing the importance of the transitions needed in the move from expert clinician to teacher of clinicians is the first step in understanding the role of teacher. The suggestions offered in this chapter provide one of the essential foundations of teaching well. The transition from clinician to teacher involves the heart, mind, body, and soul of each individual. Facilitating this process of transition is the role of the master teacher.

REFLECTIONS

Think about transition times in your own life. What made them possible and what made them positive? Can you think of a way to use transition theory and seminars in your teaching role?

REFERENCES

Adlersberg, M., & Thorne, S. (1990). Emerging from the chrysalis: Older widows in transition. *Journal of Gerontological Nursing, 16,* 4–8.

Brooten, D., Brown, L. P., Munro, B. H., York, R., Cohen, S. M., Roncoli, M., & Hollingsworth, A. (1988). Early discharge and specialist transitional care. *IMAGE: Journal of Nursing Scholarship, 20,* 64–68.

Chick, N., & Meleis, A. I. (1986). Transitions: A nursing concern. In P. L. Chinn (Ed.), *Nursing research methodology: Issues and implementation* (pp. 237–257). Rockville, MD: Aspen.

Esper, P. S. (1995). Facing transition: Nurse clinician to nurse educator. *Journal of Nursing Education, 34*(2), 89–91.

Grady, J. L. (1992). SN to GN to RN: Facilitating the transition. *Nurse Educator, 17*(4), 36, 40.

Hollander, J., & Haber, L. (1992). Ecological transition: Using Bronfenbrenner's model to study sexual identity change. *Health Care for Women International, 13,* 121–129.

MacNeil, M. (1997). From nurse to teacher: Recognizing a status passage. *Journal of Advanced Nursing, 25*(3), 634–642.

Meleis, A. I., Swayer, L. A., Im, E., Messias, D. K. H., & Schumacher, K. (2000). Experiencing transitions: An emerging middle-range theory. *Advances in Nursing Science, 23*(1), 12–28.

Mulligan, J. E. (1976). Professional transition: Nurse to nurse-midwife. *Nursing Outlook, 24*(4), 228–233.

Reed-McKay, K. L. (1989). Role transition for school nurses in the Spokane Public Schools. *Journal of School Health, 59,* 444–445.

Rice, J. M. (1988). Transition from staff nurse to head nurse: A personal experience. *Nursing Management, 19*(4), 102.

Schumacher, K. L., & Meleis, A. I. (1994). Transitions: A central concept in nursing. *IMAGE: The Journal of Nursing Scholarship, 26*(2), 119–127.

Wuest, J. (1990). Trying it on for size: Mutual support in role transition for pregnant teens and student nurses. *Health Care for Women International, 11,* 383–392.

CHAPTER 3

Ethics, Values, and Moral Development in Teaching

To be professional is to be ethical, and to practice ethically requires an understanding of ethics, values and oneself.
—J. E. Thompson and H. O. Thompson,
Bioethical Decision Making for Nurses

SUGGESTED OUTCOMES FOR THIS CHAPTER

This chapter will focus on the why, what, and how of teaching health professionals about values, ethics, moral development, and moral reasoning, and how this affective and cognitive knowledge can be applied in their professional roles. At the end of this chapter, the reader will be able to

1. discuss why it is important to bring values, morals, and ethics content to consciousness throughout the curriculum preparing advanced practice nurses and midwives;
2. define the goals of ethics teaching;
3. discuss various approaches to the teaching of ethics; and
4. understand and discuss the influence of values, moral development, moral reasoning, and ethical theories on the practice of nursing and midwifery.

INTRODUCTION

As noted in the faculty philosophy in the Preface to this book, the authors are firm believers that values and ethics must be taught rather than caught by the learners. It can be a potentially dangerous situation for a teacher to rely on personal example or modeling in the teaching of values and ethics in a professional discipline because the "gold standard" of ethical behavior and action is, at times, very difficult to sustain as a human being. We all wish to be good, to do good, to act appropriately, and to make the best decisions in our lives and in our teaching as well as in our clinical practice. There are times, however, when these ideal actions are difficult to implement.

Common sense suggests that while *modeling* moral behavior and ethical action is an honorable ideal and needed everywhere, teachers as human beings have their less than optimal moments when the stated ideal is not matched by the expected behavior, when what they say and do are not the same, thus causing potential confusion in the learner. Hence the importance of *teaching about* values, ethics, moral development, and moral reasoning as tools for understanding (knowing) expected moral behavior and ethical norms of the practice of nursing, midwifery, medicine, or any other health professional role (Holt & Long, 1999).

Education, including moral education, is rarely a onetime event—it's not as though one can put some books on a shelf, give one lecture, or lead a seminar discussion, and then the "task" of moral education is complete (Aroskar, 1977; Fry, 1986; Fry, 1989; Jameton, 1984; Thompson & Thompson, 1993). Some educators, especially in the health disciplines, call in a guest lecturer to talk "at" learners about proper professional behavior or the moral code of the profession or vague concepts like autonomy or justice, and then proceed to ignore this content in any future discussion of course content, including professional practice. The author suggests that teaching and learning about values, ethics, moral development, and moral reasoning is a life-long process and applies to teachers and learners alike. As teachers and learners we are members of a society, and as members of a society we are ethically obliged to work toward the "good" of the whole in order for that society to be maintained and to prosper. We need to understand what that "good" is and how we can promote it. We need to understand values and ethics. We need to understand how individuals develop morally as well as intellectually, and how they use critical reflection and self-knowledge to make ethical decisions in life generally and in professional practice specifically (Thompson & Thompson, 1987; Viens, 1994).

The challenge for the teacher is to facilitate the transfer and internalization of personal and professional values, morals, and ethics so that the learner uses this understanding to inform, direct, and allow them to make the best decisions in practice—to be ethical. *The goal of ethical practice is to do the right thing for the right reason* (Thompson & Thompson, 1995; Veatch & Fry, 1987).

TEACHER PREPARATION

In recognition that many nurses, midwives, and physician educators may have had limited exposure to the theoretical foundations of values, morals, and ethics in their own educational pathways, this chapter also provides a brief overview of and selected references for the content needed in this area, and suggests exercises that can be used in helping the teacher and learner understand values, levels of moral development, and the application of ethical theory to decision-making. It is also acknowledged that many health professional educators feel uneasy about teaching values and exposing values (especially personal values) to open discussion and moral discourse. They may fall into the trap of thinking that there are no "right answers" in ethics due to the pluralistic nature of our society. However, the truth in ethics education and application is that there are often many right actions or choices and the difficulty is selecting the best one for the given situation (Thompson & Thompson, 1985).

Just as any new content area can be perceived as threatening to the teacher, the best approach to becoming comfortable with the content is to study it in depth before attempting to take it to the learners. Several suggestions are offered here to assist the teacher in preparing for the task of teaching ethics. The teacher is encouraged to select a basic bioethics text and a values text—especially those written by a knowledgeable professional in their own discipline (e.g., nurse ethicist, physician ethicist, midwife ethicist, philosopher/moral theologian, etc.). Fry (1989) also suggests that reviewing the history of ethics teaching in one's discipline provides an important foundation for understanding the distinction between nursing ethics, physician ethics, midwifery ethics, etc. Some have found it helpful to begin their preparation of content with the revised edition of the *Encyclopedia of Bioethics* edited by W. T. Reich (1995). The *Encyclopedia* allows the teacher who is building his/her knowledge base in ethics to find an overview of key content areas such as ethical theory, values, moral reasoning, nursing ethics, and physician ethics, as well as some of the topical issues in the field such as genetics, informed consent, and end-of-life decision-making. Each section has an extensive bibliography that leads to further depth in understanding of the content area. In this information age, using the Internet to select some of the most recent articles in the field is also encouraged. As will be noted later in this book, one of the most important principles of teaching is that the teacher "know" the content very well so that it can be communicated to the learner in the most understandable format. This is an exciting challenge for the novice teacher in ethics, as the language of values and ethics and the almost immediate need to apply this knowledge to the care of patients require an immediate understanding.

THE "WHY" OF ETHICS TEACHING

As teachers, we are ethically obliged to create and provide the moral atmosphere in which the individual can develop as a productive member of society. "Throughout the ages, great teachers have noted life is not fully lived if it is lived only for ourselves. For fullness of life, a society needs to reach beyond itself to a higher purpose" (Thompson & Thompson, 1993, p. 3). The teaching of values, ethics, moral development, and moral reasoning, while based in the Western world on moral theology, moral philosophy, and psychology, relies on a clear understanding and sharing of insight by the teacher that goes far beyond any religious teaching or institution. Human beings are not value free—we are value-laden. Science is not value free—science is value-laden as it is carried out, discovered, and shared with others. The teaching of values and ethics, therefore, is also not value free—it is value-laden. And the values that influence what is taught in the vast arena of morality, ethics, and moral development are those deeply held values of the teacher.

The Goals of Ethics Teaching

As noted by nurse ethicist Sara T. Fry (1989), the overall goal for the teaching of ethics to nurses and other health professionals is "to produce a morally accountable practitioner who is skilled in ethical decision making." Excellent patient care results from morally insightful clinicians who are committed to making ethical decisions in their care of others and being responsible for the outcomes of those decisions. Several authors (Aroskar, 1977; Fry, 1989; Holt & Long, 1999; Krawczyk, 1997; Thompson & Thompson, 1989b) address specific objectives in ethics teaching that include offering the learner the opportunity to: 1) examine their personal commitment and values relating to the care of patients, the nature of health and illness, and human responses to one's state of health; 2) engage the learner in ethical discussion and reflection (moral discourse) based on a solid theoretical foundation; 3) develop skills in moral reasoning and moral judgment; and 4) develop the ability to use ethics knowledge for decision-making, reflect on societal issues and policy directions, and design/participate in research on the moral foundations of professional practice. The teacher must begin with stated objectives in this content area that reflect the roles and responsibilities of the health professional being taught.

THE "HOW" OF ETHICS TEACHING

The Preparation

"Know thyself" is the first step in preparing to teach values, morals, and ethics. What are the basic values that generally guide your actions and choices on a daily basis? What do you value in human relationships? What do you value about teaching? What do you value about learning? What do you value about your professional role? Are you committed to knowing your content area so well you can simplify the language and engage the learners in active discussion? These are just a few of the questions that teachers might ask themselves in preparing to teach about values and ethics. The very nature of values and valuing requires that the teacher know and willingly share personal values and biases as part of the foundation of trust that needs to be built in order for the learners to feel comfortable enough to share their own values and ethics. A trusting, respectful, and confidential environment for learning must be set and maintained by the teacher, and the expected moral behaviors must be discussed openly and modeled consistently.

Teaching Methods

There are many teaching methods that have been used for the teaching of values and ethics across and within professional disciplines. Nurse teachers, for example, began the teaching of ethics in the early decades of the 20th century based on the belief that ethics was a "science" and used a scientific model for ethics teaching that focused on the conduct and duty of nurses (Aikens, 1916; Robb, 1921). More recent views of ethics teaching include emphasis on professional codes (American Nurses Association (ANA), 1985; ACNM, 1990; International Council of Nurses (ICN), 2000; American Medical Association (AMA), 1980), values and virtues, moral development, and ethical inquiry including descriptive and normative ethical approaches to decision-making (Fry, 1989).

Contemporary methods for teaching ethics and values, especially bioethics or "life" ethics, include lecture, lecture with guided discussion, case studies with guided ethical analysis, ethics rounds, and clinical conferences with open discussion of the moral dimensions of clinical practice. Holt and Long (1999) describe the use of storytelling and a "Moot Court" for exploring the interface of ethics and law, as well providing the learner with a structured environment in which s/he can practice moral discourse, moral reasoning, and decision-making. Krawzcyk (1997) studied the development of moral judgment in nursing students measured by the Defining the Issues Test (DIT; Rest, 1993) and found that senior BSN students who had received an ethics course (42 hours) taught by a professor of ethics scored significantly higher on the DIT than those students exposed to ethics "integrated" throughout the nursing theory courses or those who had no planned ethics content in the nursing program. This is just one example of the need for health professional teachers to plan for ethics teaching, and supports the use of guided discussion and ethical inquiry within a defined time period (Cloonan et al., 1999).

The choice of teaching methods will depend on the content to be taught as well as the level of the learner. For example, the first time the teacher introduces values there are many practical exercises that can assist understanding. Steele and Harmon (1983) developed several exercises that move from the relatively simple and nonthreatening exposure of personal values to more complex thinking and reflection. Using Massey's (1981) series of videotapes on gut-level value programming is another method for understanding values that can be used fairly early in the learner's educational program. Once the learner is exposed to clinical practice in their chosen discipline, real cases from the clinical settings can be used for classroom analysis and discussion. Ethics rounds have been most successful with the advanced learner who has mastered an understanding of ethics theory and moral reasoning.

THE "WHAT" OF ETHICS TEACHING

As with any content area, the next step here is to know your content, and understand how the theoretical foundations of values, morals, moral development, and ethics can be applied to professional practice. After gaining an understanding of the theory and application of such content, make a decision on *what* you will teach *when* in the curriculum and *how* that content fits with the overall course and program of study for the learner. Selection of teaching and evaluation methods follows. The affective domain of learning is dominant in the teaching/learning of values, morals, ethics, moral development, and moral reasoning. Though this content area may seem difficult to teach at first, the rewards of learning have the potential to create wonderful health professionals.

Sequencing Content

The authors have found it effective to begin ethics teaching with values and values clarification exercises (Steele & Harmon, 1983). After examining the personal values of learners and teachers, the teacher is encouraged to then look at the values of the profession. Analysis of codes of ethics of the various disciplines (medicine, midwifery, nursing) advances the learner's understanding of the moral duties and obligations of the professional role they have chosen (Smith & Davis, 1980). Content on moral development (Kohlberg, 1984), including asking the learners to take the DIT, is then provided along with discussion of how moral development and values influence ethical/professional practice. Case studies with a values focus can be used for this area of guided discussion. This area of content consists of both descriptive ethics (describing what "is") and virtue ethics (what kind of person a nurse, midwife, physician should be) (Davis, Aroskar, Liaschenko, & Drought, 1997).

Next comes discussion of normative ethics—deontology, utilitarianism, natural law—and how this theory supports the moral justification for decision-making. At the post-baccalaureate level in health professional education, spending time on applied ethics is usually better received by learners than an overemphasis on theory—the adult learner wants to know how this theory can be used and what difference it makes in clinical care (DeCasterle et al., 1997). This learner need can best be met by using a structured model for ethical analysis of clinical cases, such as Thompson and Thompson's 10-step model in Figure 3.1 at the end of this chapter, that reinforces the need for understanding values, moral development, ethics theory, and critical reflection before jumping to a decision or conclusion (Thompson & Thompson, 1985).

Definition of Terms

When teachers and learners first approach the study and teaching of ethics, it often seems as if one is being asked to learn a new language—the language of ethics, of moral theology, of philosophy. These "languages" may be relatively new to the health professional who has spent years steeped in the language of science—of anatomy and physiology. There is little doubt, however, that the language of ethics can be learned just as health professionals learned the language of their professional practice, especially medical and nursing abbreviations that continue to confuse and obfuscate meaning for the patients they serve. Health professionals know and learn the time and dedication it takes to pay attention and use commonly understood words with the public at large rather than the language of the professional if they truly believe it is important that the public understand what it is they are trying to say or do. This same principle of using commonly understood words in teaching about values and ethics is critical to understanding the complex concepts that influence both the cognitive and affective domains of learning. The following definitions are offered to clarify the author's use of the terms before moving to how to teach others about these.

Values

Values give meaning to our lives. They are directional signals that guide our thoughts, decisions, and actions. Self-awareness is an essential ingredient for fulfilling one's professional role in health and illness care. To make ethical decisions in practice, one needs to know and understand both ethics and the personal and professional values that direct one's daily life (Thompson & Thompson, 1990b). Values help us understand what is important, what is meaningful to us and to others, what ideas or actions are worthy or appropriate or correct.

But how does one define "values"? The Latin root means to be strong, to be of worth. Other terms associated with the definition of values include prized, merit, favored, respect, regard, and appreciate. According to Raths, Harman, and Simon (1966), a value is an attitude or belief about the worth, truth or beauty of another individual, object, or action that is used to guide daily behavior or action. Steele and Harmon (1983, p. 1) defined value as "an affective disposition towards a person, object or idea" and Hall (1973) defined value as "a stance (position) that is taken and is expressed through behaviors, feelings, imagination, knowledge, and actions." There are many definitions of values with several recurring themes that formed the synthesis definition that follows.

The definition that has worked best for the author in over 25 years of teaching and learning about values is: *Values are attitudes and beliefs put into practice in our daily lives.* This definition implies a decision of what we prize or treasure enough to actually use in practice. Values clarification exercises help us to know our most deeply held values and to then more fully understand how these values influence who are we are and the decisions we make in our lives, such as choice of professional career.

Sources of Values   "Where do our values come from?" is a common question raised in the discussion of values and values clarification. The author suggests that every adult has at least three different main sources of values or value sets. These include gut-level values programmed into us during the earliest years of infancy and childhood; adult values acquired by association with individuals, groups, and causes, and through experiences that are freely chosen from alternatives; and professional values that we were socialized with during the formative years of our professional development and ongoing professional practice. Professional values are often embodied in a profession's "code of ethics" or code of moral behavior.

Looking more closely at the main sources of personal and professional values, we begin with what Morris Massey (1981) calls gut-level values. He notes that from birth to age 7, infants and children are *imprinted* with the norms of the culture—what's right, what's wrong, what's good, what's bad. The primary sources of these values include family, geography, religion, and the ever-present electronic babysitter—television. *Modeling* during the ages of 8–13 is the process for instilling gut-level values through family, education, media, economics, and peers. Peers and education also contribute to the process of *intense socialization* that further instills gut-level values during the ages of 14–20. Massey notes that nearly 90% of our gut-level values are set in place by the age of 10, hence his emphasis in self-discovery of asking adults to think about where they were when they were 10 in order to begin to understand what they were value-programmed with by family, education, economic, peers, media, religion, and geography.

Adult values are acquired in a variety of ways, primarily through socialization and choice. Simon and Clark (1975) suggest that adults acquire values that: 1) are freely chosen; 2) are chosen from alternatives; 3) require thoughtful consideration of outcomes; 4) are prized and cherished; 5) are made known to others; 6) precipitate action; and 7) are integrated into one's lifestyle. One can note the degree of free will inherent in these value theorists' view of acquiring adult values whereas gut-level values appear to be programmed into us at a very early age.

Professional values are usually acquired through socialization into the roles and responsibilities of the profession, primarily through modeling and imitation if not specifically taught in classroom and clinical sessions. Since the dominant values of the profession are often embodied in a written code of ethics or moral behavior, these codes become excellent teaching tools during the discussion of the values of the profession. Standards of practice, professional statements, and philosophies are all excellent sources of professional values. It is important to note here that gut-level values and adult and professional values often mirror one another as values and value preferences often lead to our choice of a professional career. If one's gut-level value programming is inconsistent with the values of the professional role chosen, that person often changes careers after a short period of time or elects to change their most deeply held values to adapt to the professional values.

All values can be changed, whether freely chosen or programmed in at an early age. James Rest (1979) suggests that as adults we can change our values by first recognizing a certain value, then understanding what it means for us, coming to prefer that value over others we hold, and finally making a decision to adopt that value in practice. Morris Massey (1981) suggests that gut-level values can be changed by exposure to a "significant emotional event" or what this author commonly refers to as "affective dissonance"—a situation in which at a gut level we just do not feel right about what is going on. If one acknowledges that gut-level feeling, chances are what is happening is in conflict with deeply held personal values and calls those values into consciousness. Examples of significant emotional events (SEEs) may be as dramatic as the death of a close relative or friend, loss of one's job, or divorce, or as seemingly innocuous as reading a good book or watching a movie. Whatever the stimulus, significant emotional events help bring to consciousness our most deeply held values related to life and its meaning for us. Examples of SEEs in health and illness care include negative responses to choices made by patients, families, or other team members that cause one to examine why that choice seems wrong. If such negative responses are ignored, learning can be at an impasse and the realities of clinical practice become overwhelming. On the positive side, such affective dissonance affords both teachers and learners the opportunity to examine our personal and professional values, note and understand the sources of conflict, and decide what needs changing—one's personal values, one's professional values, or one's job. Though this latter choice of changing jobs or careers may initially seem threatening to some teachers and learners, open and conscious discussion of what our profession requires of its practitioners often leads to a renewed commitment to the values of self-determination, fairness, respect for human dignity, veracity, and caring, that are core values of health professions (ANA, 1985; AMA, 1980; ACNM, 1990; ICN, 2000).

Morals

If values are directional signals for what is right or wrong, good or bad, what are morals? "Morals" comes from the Latin word *moralis* and refers to the shoulds and oughts of life, culture, society, and religion reflected in human behavior and choices. What *should* one do in this situation? What *ought* one to do or say? These are moral questions that require consideration before making a decision or choice. Morals or moral behavior goes beyond values, beyond directional signals, to action. A moral being is expected to make the right choices after thoughtful reflection and consideration of potential outcomes. Once those choices are weighed against a standard of "right" or "good" or "correctness," the moral being is expected to carry out the best choice and to be accountable for the results of his/ her behavior or action (Thompson & Thompson, 1985).

This reflective behavior and action describes what it means to be a *moral agent*—a person who is free (not coerced or intimidated) or has the power to act/ decide ("the buck stops here"). Health professionals are moral agents and need to use that power and freedom wisely. Good moral agents are committed to learning and remaining up-to-date in their professional field, to reasoning critically, to accepting responsibility for decisions and actions, and to caring for others in a manner that respects persons and human dignity (Thompson & Thompson, 1990a).

The author has found it useful to teach morals, morality, and moral development together because of the common theme of expected human behavior. When working with health professionals and teaching others to teach the next generation of health workers, it is helpful to ask them to listen for the "shoulds and oughts" in discussion of proposed treatment plans and decision-making in order to trigger their awareness of the moral dimensions of professional practice. The concept of "clinical judgment" is often a cover-up for not acknowledging the values and moral judgments being made in relation to patient care (Carlton, 1978).

If one accepts that *morals* refers to human behavior, in this case duties and obligations of health professionals, then one understands that most professional codes of *ethics* are really codes of moral behavior. This interchange of ethics and morals is common in everyday usage, but the alternative separation of ethics and morals leads to the clarity in understanding the complexity of human behavior, moral reasoning, and ethical decision-making that is required of all health professionals.

Moral Development

How one determines what should or ought to be done is based on values and levels of moral development as well as the ethical justification resulting from moral reasoning. Here the teacher needs to understand how individuals develop morally and share this insight and theory with the learner. The understanding of *moral development* can be gained from using Kohlberg's stage theory of moral development grounded in the deontological principle of justice (1984), or Gilligan's approach to moral development in women based on relationships and caring (1982), or other theorists who help one understand how we develop morally.

Important teaching points when addressing moral development include how this knowledge can expand the health professional's understanding of human behavior and how individuals make choices in their lives. For example, if the health professional is working in a "must keep at all costs" job, pre-conventional morality will be the norm as the worker does what the employer says is right out of fear of punishment (Kohlberg's Stage 1). Health professionals may understand and know a "better" alternative for action, but will not voice it out of fear of losing their employment. Likewise, a learner who fears a bad grade from a teacher may not be willing to take the risk to make principled decisions in clinical practice that would reflect post-conventional moral development (Kohlberg's Level III, Stage 6).

Using a stage theory of moral development is helpful, providing that the teacher reinforces that higher numbered stages do not mean an individual is "more moral" in their choices or actions. As Kohlberg and others have noted, most adults in a society function at a conventional level of moral development where personal authority (Stage 3) or abstract authority (the law, Stage 4) determine what is the morally correct thing to do or say. Education is strongly correlated with an individual's ability to understand and function at the higher stages of moral development (Kohlberg), as those with advanced college degrees will score higher on the Rest DIT instrument than those with less than a high school education. Thus it is reasonable to expect that learners within a professional discipline should be able to understand and function on a principled level, though we all have the capacity to function at all lower levels as well. It is also important for the health professional student to realize that they often will be viewed by patients at a conventional level of moral development as the "expert" or personal authority in many caregiving situations and asked "What should I do?" It is vital that all health professionals understand this and use their personal authority wisely. In health oriented encounters (prenatal care, family planning, etc.), the professional may take the teacher approach and help the patient make decisions about their own patterns of healthy behavior and choices. When a person is very ill, they often depend on others to make good decisions for them (substituted judgments— decisions made by others that reflect what the patient would have decided if they were capable). Whatever the situation, health professionals who understand how individuals develop morally gain insight into how individuals may respond to health or illness encounters and what will be expected of the professional.

Ethics

Any discussion of moral shoulds and oughts cannot be separated from the ethical "why" as noted in this section. If one accepts that the goal of ethical practice is to *do the right thing for the right reason*, morals are the "right thing" or action and ethics offers the explanation of the "right reason." Ethical theories provide reasons/rationale for action and choices in our lives and in the lives of patients. For many, knowing the "why" of choices helps one to evaluate the goodness of that choice. When children continually ask, "Why?"—they can be viewed as budding moral philosophers. The child's incessant questioning reflects the importance that humans place on having and understanding the reasons for what is going on. In the patient care setting, helping others make good or right choices for themselves requires the professional to know the "why" of treatment options so this rationale can be shared with the patient and increase their understanding prior to giving consent. This is the "informed" component of the ethical and legal concept of informed consent.

Ethical theories most commonly used in the Western world include utilitarianism, deonotology, and natural law (Thompson & Thompson, 1985). This chapter is not intended as a complete text on ethics, therefore a brief overview of ethics theories is offered while also directing the learner to complete texts on the subject. *Utilitarianism* supports the selection of actions or choices that will maximize the greatest happiness or "good" for the largest number of people. Utilitarian theory also can be characterized as a theory concerned primarily with good outcomes or good ends (consequences) in decision-making rather than with how (the means) one arrived at the final choice. One of the common aphorisms that summarizes the utilitarian theory is, "The end justifies the means." This is a common ethical framework for health and illness care (Thompson & Thompson, 1989a). For example, surgery (the means) is in and of itself quite hurtful (causes harm) to an individual, but when that surgery restores an individual to healthy life, it is considered a good outcome (the end). It is precisely this issue of a good end that is brought into question in illness care when surgery is proposed without hope of recovering health.

Deontology is often called the principled approach to ethical reasoning. Beauchamp and Childress (1994) several years ago offered four primary or umbrella principles for bioethics: 1) do good (beneficence), 2) do not harm (nonmaleficence), 3) self-determination (autonomy), and 4) justice (fairness). One can note the immediate relevance of these principles to decisions in health and illness care. However, there are many other deontological principles that the health professional needs to know and understand. Some of the more common ones include telling the truth (veracity), maintaining confidentiality, respect for human dignity, and non-discrimination in caregiving. Those using deontological principles to justify their moral shoulds or oughts are more concerned with the means of action rather than the ends, as opposed to the utilitarian's view. Right or moral action is based more on how the choice is made or reasoned and not so much on the expected outcome (Thompson & Thompson, 1985).

The teacher needs to help the learner understand that these principles may at times conflict with one another, such as when a family member wants "everything done to keep Mother alive" when there is little hope of recovery and Mother does not want to suffer any longer (autonomy). Paternalism or maternalism—making decisions for others when they can make those decisions for themselves—has come under severe criticism in illness care during the past 20 years as it violates the principle of self-determination. However, as noted by Woodward (1998), doing good or being beneficient in a care situation could be reasoned as ethical even though this constitutes paternalism and violates autonomy. Campbell (1994) suggests that autonomy may be viewed as the ethical ideal in our society and when a person is inappropriately dependent, the ethical challenge is to encourage "emancipation" in a sensitive and supportive manner. This suggestion reflects the importance of the human relationship in health and illness care along with the need to understand and reason morally. Using cases from clinical experiences is a helpful teaching method for identifying such conflicts and understanding the "why" of each proposed action before one is chosen.

Natural law receives minor attention in most bioethics texts. It also has many definitions, though the most common one refers to what exists in nature as the determinant of "right action." The religious prohibition against all forms of contraception (except natural ones) is often reasoned on the basis that human beings were meant to procreate and to interfere with that natural function is unethical. Natural law theory has also been used to justify the decisions made for palliative or end-of-life hospice care in that the emphasis on caregiving is to "allow nature to take its course"—to support and care for but not treat the person who is dying (Thompson & Thompson, 1989c). In general, natural law ethicists are concerned with both the means and ends of decision-making (Thompson & Thompson, 1985).

Moral Reasoning and Ethical Decision-Making

Applied ethics requires the teacher and learner to engage in moral reasoning in order to make ethical decisions. The moral reasoning process includes several discrete steps: analysis, weighing, justifying, choosing, and evaluating competing reasons for a given action. Health professionals will immediately note the similarity of these steps to the scientific process, the nursing process, or the management process used in midwifery practice (Ketefian, 1988; Thompson & Thompson,

1985). You might ask: So what is the difference? One of the major differences between the scientific method and the moral reasoning process is the emphasis in the first on science, technology, facts, etc., and the emphasis in the latter on values, moral dimensions of decision-making, and ethical justification that goes beyond science to the human core of caring for those who are ill.

Analysis helps those involved examine a given situation, clearly identify the moral dimensions of the situation and the ethical issues that they represent, and begin to consider possible choices that may be taken (alternative actions). The weighing function of moral reasoning requires that participants assess the strengths and weaknesses of each proposed action. The justifying step of moral reasoning encourages moral discourse among the key individuals in the situation and requires the reasons (ethical justification) that support each proposed action. This is often the time that values and value conflicts surface, and when one needs to understand the hierarchy of values that influence the choices about to be made. Choice of one action and immediate evaluation of the outcomes of that choice complete the process of moral reasoning or may require that another choice be made because the one chosen did not produce the desired result.

Moral reasoning should be included in all aspects of clinical decision-making, as there is a moral dimension to every patient encounter. The very nature of working with other human beings is moral. Unfortunately, clinical judgment has been used as a guise by some physicians and nurses to avoid or deny input from the patient or family, reasoning that the professional knows best (strong paternalism). Brody (1976) notes that people trained in science often try to solve ethical problems by accumulating more and more scientific data from tests. He suggests that they ignore the value dimensions of the situation and the need to make a moral judgment along with the scientific one. Until one recognizes the moral dimensions of clinical practice, ethical dilemmas that arise will not be resolved.

It is precisely the fact that health professionals need practice and support in moral reasoning and ethical justification that warrants designated time in the teaching of these professionals. The Bioethical Decision Model in Figure 3.1 has proven very helpful in analyzing the ethical dimensions of clinical practice and in teaching the influence of values, moral development, and ethical reasoning on clinical decisions. It is helpful to begin the analysis of clinical situations in the calm and safety of a classroom before proceeding to ethics rounds or an ethics committee. An atmosphere of trust, mutual respect, and a commitment to critical thinking and moral reasoning are the basic requirements for using the decision model. The outcome of such learning and moral discourse is better patient care for all.

REFLECTIONS

Think about where you were when you were ten years old and reflect on the values you received from family, friends, religion, media (books, television, Internet), geographic location, and social status. How many of these values guide your life today as a professional? How might these values affect your teaching and work with learners from different backgrounds, ages, or races? To what extent have you internalized the code of ethics (moral behavior) of nursing and your professional specialty? What type of information do you need to establish a level of competence and confidence in teaching values, morals, and ethics to advanced practice nurses and midwives? Develop a personal plan for obtaining this information.

SUGGESTED EXERCISES

1.   Work with a group (no more than 10–12) of colleagues to select patient care scenarios that can be used with the Bioethical Decision Model (Figure 3.1).

Step One: **Review the situation** to determine health problems, decision/actions needed, ethical components, and key individuals and relative priority of each.

Step Two: **Gather additional information** to clarify the situation and understand: why that information is needed (values); legal constraints, if any; and other constraints such as time, lack of decision capacity, institutional policies.

Step Three: **Identify the ethical issues or concerns in the situation**; explore the historical roots, current philosophical/religious positions, and societal views on each issue.

Step Four: **Define personal and professional moral positions** on the issues/concerns identified in Step Three, including a review of personal constraints raised by the issues and professional code(s) for guidance (e.g., ANA, AMA, ACNM). Identify conflicting loyalties/obligations, and level of moral development operant.

Step Five: **Identify moral positions** of key individuals in situation as well as level of moral development when possible.

Step Six: **Identify value conflicts**, if any, and attempt to understand the basis for conflict, possible resolution, and whether outside help is needed.

Step Seven: **Determine who should make the needed decision** and your specific role in the situation.

Step Eight: **Identify the range of actions** with anticipated outcomes for each, including moral justification, and then decide which action/decision fits the situation.

Step Nine: **Decide on a course of action and carry it out**; know the reasons for the choice of action/decision, be able to explain reasons to others, and establish a time frame for review of outcomes.

Step Ten: **Evaluate/review results of decision-making**, including determining whether the expected outcome occurred, whether a new decision is needed, and whether the decision process was complete.

FIGURE 3.1   Bioethical Decision Model.

Adapted from Thompson and Thompson (1985).

Practice applying the decision model and evaluate each step of the process as well as the group's determination of the appropriate use of the decision model.

2. Work as a group of teachers to develop a code of moral behavior for teachers of advanced practice nurses and midwives. Share this code with learners along with the learner code of behavior of the university (usually a code of academic integrity or honor code). Discuss with learners how these codes of moral behavior overlap and where they are different, if so.

REFERENCES

ACNM. (1990). *Code of ethics for nurse-midwives.* Washington, DC: ACNM.

Aikens, C. A. (1916). *Studies in ethics for nurses.* Philadelphia: W. B. Saunders Co.

American Medical Association. (1980). *Principles of medical ethics.* Chicago: Author.

American Nurses Association. (1978). *Perspectives on the code for nurses.* Kansas City, MO: Author.

American Nurses Association. (1985). *Code for nurses with interpretive statements.* Kansas City, MO: Author.

Aroskar, M. A. (1977). Ethics in the nursing curriculum. *Nursing Outlook, 25,* 260–264.

Beauchamp, T., & Childress, J. (1994). *Principles of biomedical ethics.* Oxford, United Kingdom: Oxford University Press.

Brody, H. (1976). *Ethical decisions in medicine.* Boston: Little, Brown.

Campbell, A. V. (1994). *Moderate love: A theology of professional care.* London: The Society for Promoting Christian Knowledge.

Carlton, W. (1978). *In our professional opinion: The primacy of clinical judgement over moral choice.* Notre Dame: University of Notre Dame Press.

Cloonan, P. A., Davis, F. D., & Burnett, C. B. (1999). Interdisciplinary education in clinical ethics: A work in progress. *Holistic Nursing Practice, 13*(2), 12–19.

Davis, A. J., Aroskar, M. A., Liaschenko, J., & Drought, T. S. (1997). *Ethical dilemmas and nursing practice* (4th ed.). Stamford, CT: Appleton & Lange.

DeCasterle, B., Gryponck, M., Vuylsteke-Wauters, M., & Janssen, P. (1997). Nursing students' responses to ethical dilemmas in nursing practice. *Nursing Ethics, 4*(1), 12–28.

Fry, S. T. (1986). Ethical inquiry in nursing: The state of the art. *Virginia Nurse, 54,* 12–13.

Fry, S. T. (1989). Teaching ethics in nursing curricula. *Nursing Clinics of North America, 24*(2), 485–497.

Gilligan, C. (1982). *In a different voice: Psychological theory and women's development.* Cambridge, MA, and London: Harvard University Press.

Hall, B. P. (1973). *Value clarification as a learning process.* New York: Paulist Press.

Holt, J., & Long, T. (1999). Moral guidance, moral philosophy, and moral issues in practice. *Nurse Education Today, 19*(3), 246–249.

International Council of Nurses. (2000). *ICN code for nurses.* Geneva, Switzerland: Author.

Jameton, A. (1984). *Nursing practice: The ethical issues.* Englewood Cliffs, NJ: Prentice-Hall.

Ketefian, S. (1988). *Moral reasoning and ethical practice in nursing: An integrative review.* New York: National League for Nursing.

Kohlberg, L. (1984). *Essays on moral development: The psychology of moral development.* New York: Harper and Row.

Krawczyk, R. M. (1997). Teaching ethics: Effect on moral development. *Nursing Ethics, 4*(1), 57–65.

Massey, M. (1981). *What you are is . . .* [Film series]. (Available from Farmington Hills, MI: Magnetic Video).

Raths, L. E., Harmin, M., & Simon, S. B. (1966). *Values and teaching.* Columbus, OH: Merrill.

Reich, W. T. (1995). *Encyclopedia of bioethics.* New York: Simon & Schuster MacMillan.

Rest, J. R. (1979). *Development in judging moral issues.* Minneapolis: University of Minnesota Press.

Rest, J. R. (1993). *Guide for the Defining Issues Test.* Minneapolis: Center for the Study of Ethical Development.

Robb, I. H. (1921). *Nursing ethics: For hospital and private use.* Cleveland: E. C. Loeckert.

Simon, S. B., & Clark, J. (1975). *Beginning values clarification.* San Diego: Pennant.

Smith, S. J., & Davis, A. J. (1980). Ethical dilemmas: Conflicts among rights, duties and obligations. *American Journal of Nursing, 80*(8), 1463–1466.

Steele, S., & Harmon, V. (1983). *Values clarification in nursing* (2nd ed.). Norwalk, CT: Appleton-Century-Crofts.

Thompson, H. O., & Thompson, J. E. (1987). Toward a professional ethic. *Journal of Nurse-Midwifery, 32*(2), 105–109.

Thompson, H. O., & Thompson, J. E. (1993). *Moral development and moral education.* New Delhi: Indian Society for Promoting Christian Knowledge.

Thompson, J. E., & Thompson, H. O. (1985). *Bioethical decision making for nurses.* Norwalk, CT: Appleton-Century-Crofts.

Thompson, J. E., & Thompson, H. O. (1989a). Let's be practical. *Neonatal Network, 7*(6), 84–85.

Thompson, J. E., & Thompson, H. O. (1989b). Moral development. *Neonatal Network, 8*(2), 69–70.

Thompson, J. E., & Thompson, H. O. (1989c). Nature's way. *Neonatal Network, 8*(1), 93–94.

Thompson, J. E., & Thompson, H. O. (1990a). Sources of moral authority: What is right? *Neonatal Network, 8*(5), 77–79.

Thompson, J. E., & Thompson, H. O. (1990b). Values: Directional signals for life choices. *Neonatal Network, 8*(4), 83–84.

Thompson, J. E., & Thompson, H. O. (1995). *Handbook of ethics for midwives.* Philadelphia: University of Pennsylvania School of Nursing.

Veatch, R. M., & Fry, S. T. (1987). *Case studies in nursing ethics.* Philadelphia: JB Lippincott Company.

Viens, D. C. (1994). Moral dilemmas experienced by nurse practitioners. *Nurse Practitioner Forum, 5*(4), 209–214.

Woodward, V. M. (1998). Caring, patient autonomy and the stigma of paternalism. *Journal of Advanced Nursing, 28*(5), 1046–1052.

CHAPTER 4

Educational Philosophy and Adult Learning Theories

We do not think of the ordinary person as preoccupied with such difficult and profound questions as: What is truth? What is authority? To whom do I listen? What counts for me as evidence? How do I know? Yet to ask ourselves these questions and to reflect on our answers is more than an intellectual exercise, for our basic assumptions about the nature of truth and reality and the origins of knowledge shape the way we see the world and ourselves as participants in it. They affect our definitions of ourselves, the way we interact with others, our public and private personae, our sense of control over life events, our views of teaching and learning, and our conceptions of morality.

—M. F. Belenky, B. M. Clinchy, N. R. Goldberger, and
J. M. Tarule, *Women's Ways of Knowing:*
The Development of Self, Voice and Mind

SUGGESTED OUTCOMES FOR THIS CHAPTER

At the completion of this chapter the reader should be able to

1. analyze how philosophy and values influence the teaching/learning process;
2. describe the value of learning theories; and
3. compare and contrast learning theories in relation to their view of the learning process, the purpose of education, and the role of the teacher.

DEVELOPING A PHILOSOPHY OF EDUCATION

A philosophy of education considers who is to be educated, what the goals of the educational process are, what the appropriate means are to achieve those goals, and how we can evaluate the effectiveness of the teaching. When clearly delineated it provides a structure for the entire educational process. Developing and articulating a clear philosophy of education requires thoughtful consideration of your own beliefs, an understanding of research done in the field, and a willingness to be open to new ideas. Formulating your own philosophy of education should be the first step in the process of becoming an educator. Once completed it is not a document that remains filed safely in a desk. Review, clarification, and reconsideration of the philosophy you develop should happen frequently. As you build teaching experience, as research uncovers new insights in the teaching/learning process, and as the roles of advanced practice nurses (APNs) and midwives evolve it is important to consider whether this new knowledge challenges any of your previous beliefs or values.

Unfortunately, philosophy is often considered an impractical, theoretical discipline with little relevance to the "real world." However, philosophy permeates all of our lives and "raises questions about what we do and why we do it" (Elias & Merriam, 1980, p. 5). It is not an impractical, mental exercise, rather it "inspires one's activities and gives direction to practice" (Elias & Merriam, 1980, p. 5). It attempts to answer the following three questions: What is real? How do we know? What is of value? (Apps, 1973).

All of us have a rationale for our actions in any particular situation. This rationale is made up of our beliefs about the need to act, the appropriateness of the action, and the desired or anticipated result of acting. We may or may not be conscious of these beliefs; nevertheless, they will drive our actions. Combined, these beliefs make up our personal philosophy of life. Some components of our philosophy of life are our values and beliefs about individuals, society, nursing, and education. Often, we are not consciously aware of many of these values and beliefs and their impact on our approach to teaching and learning.

Because our beliefs have such a powerful influence over our actions it is important when considering a role as a teacher that we identify and analyze our beliefs about teaching and learning. Some of our beliefs may be inconsistent. Through careful thought, inconsistencies and incompletely formulated ideas can be identified and clarified, leading to a logical and organized beginning philosophy of education. Beginning the process of developing a working philosophy of education can be confusing, bringing to mind such questions as where to begin and what to include. Elias and Merriam (1980), well-known educators, provide us with areas to consider. They suggest examining our beliefs about " . . . the aims and objectives of education, curriculum or subject matter, general methodological principles, analysis of the teaching-learning process, and the relationship between education and the society in which education takes place" (p. 5).

King (1986) offers some ideas to provide structure when considering a philosophy specific to nursing education. She urges consideration of the following: the nature of nursing; the role of nurses in the health care system; the purpose of education; the nature of learning, teaching, and of education for the practice of nursing; the professional values in nursing; individual differences in learner abilities and learner styles; and the rights of the learner and the rights of the teacher. For educators who are concerned about the preparation of APNs it is important to consider your beliefs about the education of adults, the role of APNs, their scope of practice, collegiality in health care, and access to health care. See Appendix A for a sample educational philosophy, the philosophy of education to which the authors of this text ascribe.

In addition to clarifying your own individual philosophy of education it is important to compare it with the educational philosophy of the institution in which you will be teaching, and the philosophy of faculty members with whom you will be associated. It is essential that there is a philosophical match among faculty members and between faculty and the university. Additionally, prospective students should be informed of the philosophy of the institution, program, and faculty, and they should be encouraged to consider it in their selection of an educational institution. A mismatch of philosophies can be a reason for confusion among students, disagreements among faculty, and dissatisfaction with the teaching role.

LEARNING THEORIES

Learning theories are based on the educational philosophy of the theorist. They represent the practical application of an individual's beliefs about learning and represent an attempt to explain how learning occurs. They are much more detailed than an educational philosophy in how to approach the teaching/learning encounter. Some doubt the usefulness of studying learning theories but they provide us with a variety of ways for us to think about learning. In addition, they can provide a vocabulary for us to use when discussing teaching/learning. They can serve as a conceptual framework, which suggests what we should keep in mind when considering teaching/learning. Over time a number of individuals have very carefully articulated their beliefs about what learning is. Generally, these learning theories fall within four general categories: behaviorist, cognitive, humanist, and social learning.

As we describe these theories you will easily see how a philosophy of education drives a learning theory. For example, if one of your educational beliefs is that the outcome of learning is the ability of individuals to realize and achieve their potential then you would not subscribe to the behaviorist or cognitive school of learning theories.

Behaviorist Theory

Behaviorists believe that successful learning is characterized by a change in observable behavior rather than an internal thought process. This change in behavior occurs when a link or connection is made between two events—a stimulus and a response. By manipulation of this link, behavior can be changed. Learning occurs as a response to a stimulus that is repeated and reinforced. A number of individuals have presented variations on the behaviorist approach to learning. Perhaps the most well known is Pavlov who developed the theory of classical conditioning. Most are familiar with his experiments on salivation in dogs. Pavlov would ring a bell each time he presented meat powder to dogs. After conditioning, the dogs would salivate when the bell was rung regardless of whether or not food was presented at the same time. The dogs had "learned" a response to the sound of the bell and this response was observable (Bigge & Shermis, 1999; Cust, 1995; Elias & Merriam, 1980; McKenna, 1995a).

Another well-known behavioral theorist, Thorndike, further developed the theory by suggesting that learning occurred when a specific response became linked to a specific stimulus, the S-R theory of learning. He believed that if the outcome of the response were positive then the response would be repeated. He labeled this the "law of effect"—satisfying results serve to strengthen the stimulus-response link. He also proposed two other laws of learning. The "law of exercise" states that repetition of the stimulus and response results in learning and the "law of readiness" states that the learner must be ready for the connection—if not, learning is inhibited (Bigge & Shermis, 1999; Elias & Merriam, 1980; Merriam & Caffarella, 1991; McKenna, 1995a).

Building on Thorndike's work, Skinner developed the principle of "operant conditioning." This principle states that behavior is directed by its consequences and is directed toward certain desirable objectives. Positive reinforcement of the behavior ensures its continuance. Punishment can be used to eliminate or decrease a behavior (Merriam & Caffarella, 1991).

A number of educational practices are based on the behaviorist approach to learning; programmed learning, behavioral objectives, competency-based education, computer assisted instruction, mastery learning, and contract learning (Elias & Merriam, 1980; Merriam & Cafferella, 1991). The behaviorist approach to learning has characterized much of nursing education, particularly the teaching of psychomotor skills. Tasks have been taught based on measurable learning objectives, delineated procedures, simple steps, and observable outcomes. The content and structure is completely determined by the teacher (Dignam, 1992).

Cognitive Theory

Cognitivists believe that learning is an internal purposive process concerned with thinking, perception, organization, and insight. Learning is meaningful if it is connected to concepts. Unlike behaviorists, cognitivists believe that learning is not directly observable but is an internal process. In this process the learner is actively involved in problem solving, seeking out new information, and drawing on past experience in order to gain understanding. Successful learning is demonstrated as understanding and skilled performance. We can trace cognitive theory all the way back to Plato and his belief that physical objects have corresponding abstract forms that we come to know through reflection. Much of the cognitivists' work is based on German psychologists' perception of Gestalt. Gestalt theory of learning proposes that learning occurs through insight. In insightful learning the learner solves problems by constructing a new whole from individual parts. This learning is transferable and repeated in similar situations. Previous experience or knowledge is adapted to form new insights. It is believed that the individual learns from seeing the whole rather than breaking something down in parts (Cust, 1995; McKenna, 1995b; Merriam & Caffarella, 1991).

Bruner, one of the most well-known cognitivists, developed a theory of learning through discovery. Discovery learning relies on a frame of reference, which he calls a system of representation, that gives meaning to experiences. This frame of reference consists of three modes: enactive, iconic, and symbolic. In the enactive mode there exists a habitual set of actions that the learner knows without words or imagery. Often this enactive mode consists of psychomotor skills. The learner may not know the rationale or meaning behind the skill. A child's ability to ride a bike is an example of the enactive mode. The iconic mode is based on imagery. The image represents a concept but doesn't completely define it. The symbolic mode moves the iconic mode image into a symbolic system, usually language (Bigge & Shermis, 1999; Bruner, 1966; Merriam & Caffarella, 1991).

Ausubel, another well-known cognitivist, was concerned with a learner's ability to assimilate new knowledge into their already existing conceptual structure. He presented the concept of using an "advanced organizer," a general statement to be introduced about the subject that serves to organize the learner's thoughts prior to introducing detailed content about the subject. He believed that this advanced organizer would allow the student to have a frame of reference for the new knowledge and connect it to pre-existing knowledge (Ausubel, 1968; Merriam & Caffarella, 1991).

The cognitivist approach to nursing education can be seen in the selection and use of experiences to specifically develop problem solving abilities, abstract thinking, and reflective practice. All of the control of the teaching/learning experience remains with the teacher (Dignam, 1992).

Humanist Theory

Humanist theorists are concerned with feelings and experiences and the human potential for growth. They base much of their work on Maslow's hierarchy of needs and theory of motivation, and believe that education should lead to personal growth, personal fulfillment, and the achievement of self-actualization (Dignam, 1992; McKenna, 1995c; Merriam & Cafarella, 1991; Purdy, 1977).

Rogers further developed humanist theory and believed that significant meaningful educational experiences must involve the whole person, be self-initiated, make a difference in the behavior and attitudes of the learner, be evaluated by the learner, and have meaning for the learner. He advocates a student-centered approach to learning where the learners are free to determine their learning needs and to direct their own learning. There can be minimal requirements and curricular limits but the process of fulfilling the curriculum requirements is free. This learner-driven approach stems from Rogers's belief that individuals have a potential for growth and strive to better themselves (Dignam, 1992; McKenna, 1995; Merriam & Cafarella, 1991). With humanist learning theory, power lies with the learner. For success it requires a well-motivated learner (Dignam, 1992).

Adult Learning Theory

Malcolm Knowles followed Rogers's thinking and developed the theory of andragogy, a theory of adult learning. He believes that because adults come to the learning experience with a vast amount of previous knowledge and experience, the usual pedagogical methods of teaching are inappropriate and the learner should be allowed to be self-directing, even helping to formulate the curriculum (Dignam, 1992; McKenna, 1995; Merriam & Cafarella, 1991).

His theory presented a new approach to the education of adults that has become one of the best known in the field. Andragogy is based on a number of assumptions about adult learners: (a) adults, as they mature, move from the dependency of childhood to self-direction; (b) over time individuals accumulate an increasing reservoir of experience that is a valuable resource for them and others during the learning process; (c) adults are ready to learn when real life tasks or problems require new knowledge or skills; (d) adults want to be able to apply what they learn immediately and in real life situations.

Several implications for teachers flow from these assumptions about how adults learn best: (a) adults should be respected for the previous experiences they have had and a spirit of mutuality should exist between teacher and student, (b) teachers should assist learners in the self-diagnosis of learning needs, (c) learners should be involved in planning how their learning needs will be met, (d) the teacher is a guide who helps another learn rather than being an instructor in charge of teaching and learning, (e) teachers assist learners to gather evidence about the progress they are making toward their goals, (f) the evaluation process is mutual as the learner and teacher also evaluate how well the program assisted the learner in achieving those goals.

These assumptions also will drive the types of learning experiences that will have more meaning for the adult learner. Group discussions, case studies, simulations, role-playing, and seminars will all tap into the adult's reservoir of experience. In addition, providing learning experiences that help learners plan how to apply their learning to their everyday experiences will have meaning for adult learners (Knowles, 1984).

Emancipatory Education

One branch of humanist theory is referred to as emancipatory education. It views the purpose of education as a transforming experience that empowers the learner. Two contemporary and well-known theorists are associated with this school of thought.

Mezirow introduced the theory of critical reflection in learning. He defines learning as "the process of making a new or revised interpretation of the meaning of an experience, which guides subsequent understanding, appreciation, and action"(Mezirow, 1985, p. 1). This process is often stimulated by a disorienting dilemma such as death of a loved one, divorce, or retirement. These dilemmas require one to reexamine beliefs about self and the future.

Mezirow identifies two dimensions in making meaning: schemes and perspectives. Schemes are sets of expected relationships, such as food satisfies hunger, or running is faster than walking. Perspectives are higher order schemes. They refer to "the structure of assumptions within which new experience is assimilated and transformed by one's past experience during the process of interpretation" (Mezirow, 1985, p. 2). Most meaning perspectives are acquired during childhood through cultural assimilation and socialization but some are learned intentionally. As adults we reflect back on prior learning to determine whether what we have just learned is congruent with our previous meaning perspectives or justified by current circumstances. Critical reflection is the term used by Mezirow to describe challenging the validity of presuppositions in prior learning. Reflective interpretation is the process of correcting distortions in our reasoning and attitudes. Perspective transformation, the result of learning, is "the process of becoming critically aware of how and why our presuppositions have come to constrain the way we perceive, understand, and feel about our world; of reformulating these assumptions to permit a more inclusive, discriminating, permeable, and integrative perspective; and of making decisions or otherwise acting upon these new understandings" (Mezirow, 1985, p. 14).

Paulo Freire, a Latin American educator, espouses a radical form of adult education in which the true function of education is radical conscientization among the oppressed. He believes that education is a potentially liberating and emancipatory process. Education promotes critical reflection, which informs action and brings about change. His theory proposes using education to bring about social, political, and economic changes in society (Elias & Merriam, 1980; Freire, 1973; Purdy, 1997a, 1997b).

Social Learning Theory

A more contemporary psychologist and learning theorist, Albert Bandura, developed the theory of social learning. This theory posits that individuals can learn not only by performing in the stimulus-response arena, as behaviorists believe, but also by observing the behavior of others and its consequences. Learning can occur not only through the individual's experience but also through observing the experience of others without having to imitate that experience of others. Observational learning is influenced by four factors: attention, retention, behavioral rehearsal, and motivation. His theory contains a reciprocal concept—people influence their environment, which then influences the way they behave. Learning is set within a social context (Merriam & Caffarella, 1991).

THE APPLICATION OF LEARNING THEORY TO APN AND MIDWIFERY EDUCATION

Students who enter an APN or midwifery program of education are clearly adults. We believe that the application of adult learning theory to their education is imperative. You may have noted as we have that many learners come to us after a disorienting life event, like marriage, divorce, or the death of a loved one. Mezirow sees these life events as often being the stimulus for beginning the process of perspective transformation. In addition, the role change from nursing practice to advanced nursing practice will require a reconsideration of the learner's beliefs and values. Our learners must examine their beliefs about the role of nurses and nurses' participation and influence in the area of health care and health care policy. For many learners, seeing the nurse as an independent practitioner who assumes total responsibility for the care of a patient is a new and frightening concept. Truly, in advanced practice, "the buck stops here," with the APN and midwife. APNs often practice alone or with a few colleagues, outside the structure of the hospital setting, outside the protection of institutional policies and procedures, and without immediate access to another professional's opinion or assistance. Learners must reconcile this role with their personal philosophy of nursing, women's roles, health care, health access, and any number of other beliefs. The discomfort, which results from challenging previously held beliefs about self or role are often manifested in learner behavior. The angry or hostile learner, the challenging learner, and the disruptive learner may be experiencing the discomfort of changing long held beliefs. Movement toward autonomy and self-direction often involves threatening elements. Overreaction to small issues often gives an indication of the degree of anxiety experienced by learners as they move toward a new concept of self. We believe that adult educational theory takes into consideration the complexity of adult learning and respects the difficulty with which learners change long held beliefs in an attempt to integrate new knowledge and skills.

One important aspect of APN and midwifery education is the examination of issues of justice and ethics in our current health care system. We believe as Friere does that the education of APNs and midwives should result in their addressing of social, political, and economic forces that contribute to the inequalities which exist in our health care system and our society as a whole. Furthermore we believe that as a result of their education APNs and midwives in turn will use the process of conscientization with their clients in an attempt to liberate them from the societal inequities that compromise their health.

Adhering to adult learning theory does not mean that we disregard teaching techniques based on sound data that are more central to other schools of thought. We must adjust those activities for adult learners. For example, we know that repetition is important in learning a psychomotor skill. The difference between a teacher with an adult learning theoretical approach and the teacher with a behaviorist approach is that, for the former, the number of repetitions necessary for mastery would not be determined solely by the teacher. In an adult education theory approach the number and timing of repetitions would be a mutual decision between teacher and learner.

REFLECTIONS

Recall your very best learning experience. Think about the factors that contributed to making that experience positive as they related to the teacher, the learner, the content of the experience, and the environment. Some questions to consider are: What learning theories did the teacher appear to embrace; how did that affect the experience? What type of learner were you—active or passive? How did other learners contribute to the experience? How did you feel about yourself during the experience?

REFERENCES

Apps, J. (1973). *Toward a working philosophy of adult education.* Syracuse, New York: Eric Clearinghouse on Adult Education.

Ausubel, D. P. (1968). *Educational psychology: A cognitive view*. New York: Holt, Rinehart and Winston.

Belenky, M. F., Clinchy, B. M., Goldberger, N. R., & Tarule, J. M. (1986). *Women's ways of knowing: The development of self, voice and mind*. New York: Basic Books.

Bigge, M. L., & Shermis, S. (1999). *Learning theories for teachers*. New York: Addison Wesley Longman, Inc.

Bruner, J. S. (1966). *Towards a theory of instruction*. Cambridge, MA: Harvard University Press.

Cust, J. (1995). Recent cognitive perspectives on learning—implications for nurse education. *Nursing Education Today, 15*(4), 280–290.

Dignam, D. (1992). Cinderella and the four learning theories. *Nursing Praxis in New Zealand, 7*(3), 17–20.

Elias, J. L., & Merriam, S. (1980). *Philosophical foundations of adult education*. Huntington, NY: Krieger Publishing Company.

Friere, P. (1973). *Education for critical consciousness*. New York: Seabury.

King, I. (1986). *Curriculum and instruction in nursing: Concepts and process*. Norwalk, CT: Appleton-Century Crofts.

Knowles, M. (1984). *Andragogy in action*. San Francisco: Jossey-Bass.

McKenna, G. (1995a). Learning theories made easy: Behaviourism. *Nursing Standard, 9*(29), 28–31.

McKenna, G. (1995b). Learning theories made easy: Cognitivism. *Nursing Standard, 10*(30), 25–28.

McKenna, G. (1995c). Learning theories made easy: Humanism. *Nursing Standard, 9*(31), 29–31.

Merriam, S., & Caffarella, R. (1991). *Learning in adulthood*. San Francisco: Jossey-Bass.

Mezirow, J. (1985). *Fostering critical reflection in adulthood*. San Francisco: Jossey-Bass.

Purdy, M. (1997a). Humanist ideology and nurse education: Humanist educational theory. *Nurse Education Today, 17*, 192–195.

Purdy, M. (1997b). Humanist ideology and nurse education: Limitations of humanist educational theory in nurse education. *Nurse Education Today, 17*, 196–202.

CHAPTER 5

Critical Thinking

... over the years I felt with increasing urgency that if education were to make any real difference in their lives, my students had to learn how to think for themselves ...
—L. A. Daloz, *Effective Teaching and Mentoring*

SUGGESTED OUTCOMES FOR THIS CHAPTER

At the end of this chapter, the reader, with practice, will be able to

1. define and discuss the concept of critical thinking as distinct from ordinary thinking and problem solving;
2. explore critical thinking attitudes and traits and their effects on clinical decision-making;
3. recognize and explain the limitations of critical thinking in advanced practice nursing and midwifery;
4. select teaching methods in the classroom and clinical areas that support and foster critical thinking in others;
5. list several teacher behaviors that will help learners to think critically about content they are learning and their provision of health care to others; and
6. define the criteria for making good decisions in clinical practice.

INTRODUCTION

This chapter is devoted to a discussion of thinking about thinking and how to improve our thinking skills. How do we think? How did humans learn to think?

What facilitates thinking and what interferes with thinking? Is there a difference in just thinking and "critical" thinking? These are just a few of the questions raised when one begins to think about thinking and how to teach others to think critically. As noted in the quote above, one of the primary challenges of any teacher is to foster thinking in the learner—to encourage, cajole, infect, and to reward all efforts in thinking that lead to understanding, reflection, and good decisions in life as well as in one's professional discipline. The Socratic method of teaching can facilitate thoughtful reflection and individual thinking and is often held in high esteem by teachers, but not even this teaching method will be successful if the learner chooses not to think independently. Intellectual, psychological, and moral maturity are required for critical thinking, but these can be diminished by environmental factors and teacher behaviors that impede another's ability to think in a critical manner.

Setting the stage for thinking and reflection is the primary responsibility of the teacher. This begins with the understanding that critical thinking is more than a cognitive process—it has a strong affective dimension as well. Likewise, the teacher needs to understand that critical thinking is *not* synonymous with problem solving or clinical judgment or scientific processing (Gordon, 2000; Scheffer & Rubenfeld, 2000; Tanner, C. A., 2000). Modeling good thinking skills for learners is very important, as is allowing learners the opportunities to think, to reflect, to make mistakes, and to learn from those errors in thinking.

In clinical disciplines such as nursing and midwifery, critical thinking is essential for good patient care. Much to the dismay of novice learners, there is no one recipe for taking care of individuals seeking health and illness services. Each individual brings their own set of concerns, expectations, symptoms, and needs to the health professional who then must listen, sort, prioritize, discuss, and plan for care, together with the patient. As midwives usually learn early in their career, no one pregnancy is the same and no labor and birth are exactly the same. It even appears at times that what one studies and learns about anatomy and physiology may be different from one body to the next. Likewise, it is evident that most newborns did not read the obstetric text defining the mechanisms of labor, as their path to birth did not always follow those mechanisms. When faced with the unexpected or the unknown, one needs to think quickly, reflect wisely, and proceed to action based on new information. Thinking is the basis for everything nurses and midwives do, and learning how to think critically and using that critical thinking process is crucial to the practice of these professions. This has led some midwifery teachers to characterize critical thinking as having three essential components or responsibilities: detective, reflective, and effective (Hunter & Lops, 1994).

TEACHER PREPARATION

For the teacher preparing to teach others about critical thinking and "how to do it" there are many excellent articles and books on the topic. One of the newest and easiest texts to use is by Green (2000), in which the author briefly reviews the history of emphasis on critical thinking in nursing, summarizes key points on critical thinking from various authors in the field, and then offers the teacher a variety of case studies that can be used across the curriculum. It is recommended that the teacher balance this summary of critical thinking with primary sources that include well-known writers in the field of critical thinking, including non-nurses and nurses, such as Alfaro-LeFevre (1995), Perry (1970), Paul (1990), Ennis (1985), Facione and Facione (1994), Bandman and Bandman (1988), Oermann (1998), and Daly (1998), as well as writers in the various specialties of advanced practice nursing like Harbison (1991), Hunter and Lops (1994), and Scheffer and Rubenfeld (2000). An extended bibliography is offered at the end of this chapter and the teacher is also encouraged to monitor current journals for articles and new approaches to the understanding and use of critical thinking in the health disciplines drawn from both nursing and non-nursing sources.

DEFINITIONS OF CRITICAL THINKING

There are several writers who offer definitions of critical thinking and whose definitions have been used to develop instruments for evaluating the use of critical thinking in learners. Robert Ennis (1985) defines critical thinking as reflective, and reasonable thinking as focused on what to do or believe. Richard Paul (1990) defines critical thinking as self-directed, disciplined thinking that demonstrates the best of thinking and mastery of intellectual skills and abilities. Bandman and Bandman (1995) define critical thinking as a rational investigation of ideas, inferences, assumptions, principles, arguments, conclusions, issues, beliefs, and actions that covers scientific reasoning, the nursing process, decision-making, and reasoning in controversial issues. Many of these authors go on to discuss the attitudes or traits of the mind required for critical thinking. Some of these will be reviewed later.

Given that there are many definitions of critical thinking in the literature, with many common themes, the authors of this text have adopted the following definition of critical thinking. *Critical thinking is an affective and cognitive process that combines the art of reason and logic with reflection, feelings, and values in order to challenge assumptions, acknowledge the unknown or unexpected, and make decisions—based on sound rationale—that lead to action.* Critical thinking is a process, not just a one time event. In other words, it is a rational approach to seeking information combined with reflection, analysis, and decision-making. Critical thinking means being prepared for the unknown, the unexpected, the different. It requires a willingness to think and to be responsible for the outcomes of that thinking.

The authors' experience with critical thinking in advanced nursing and midwifery practice supports the notions of reflection, reasoning, and exploration of the unknown and unexpected before decision-making that goes beyond the nursing process (Bandman & Bandman, 1988), the scientific method (Kataoka-Yahiro & Sayor, 1994), or the nurse-midwifery management process (Hunter & Lops, 1994). In fact, early nursing writings on the topic of critical thinking conceptualized this form of thinking as problem solving or the nursing process (Gordon, 2000). Jones and Brown (1991) conducted a survey of deans and directors of National League for Nursing (NLN) accredited schools of nursing and found support of their hypothesis: "The predominant model in baccalaureate nursing education in the United States is predicated on critical thinking as a problem solving activity, using principles of objectivity, prediction and control" (p. 529). While problem solving is vital to the provision of health and illness care, it is important to impress upon the adult learners that objectivity, prediction, and control of patient care situations are not always possible nor desirable.

Ford and Profetto-McGrath (1994) suggest that defining critical thinking solely as problem solving lends a "technical" approach to nursing practice and curriculum rather than an emancipatory approach to curriculum as praxis based on critical reflection and a more egalitarian teacher/learner relationship. This egalitarian approach to teaching and learning is very much in keeping with the principles of adult learning espoused by Knowles and associates (1984) and others (see chapter 4). Ford and Profetto-McGrath note that "to think critically and reflectively is to go beneath the surface structure of the situation, to reveal the underlying assumptions that constrain open discourse and autonomous and responsible action" (p. 343). As noted by Shor and Freire (1987), reflection illuminates reality and can change our understanding and perception of the situation. It allows us to view the situation within its context and to view new possibilities. Such reflection is vital to advanced practice nursing and midwifery care, as the very nature of that care is about relationships, values, and the meaning of health or the experience of sickness for both provider and patient/family (Phillips, 2000).

There are two distinct aspects of critical reflection (Ford & Profetto-McGrath, 1994) that have impact on the provision of quality health or illness care. The first requires a critical examination of one's own practice—including such questions as: Am I meeting standards? Do I have up-to-date knowledge and understanding of my role and expectations? Do I know what I am doing and what needs to be done in this situation? The other aspect of critical reflection requires an understanding of the situation and the way the system works to maintain the status quo (organizational values and knowledge; Schon, 1983). Critical self-reflection requires an examination of the basis for one's clinical practice along with an understanding of how one perceives the situation at hand. Krejci (1997) suggests the use of guided imagery to explore mental models, unconscious or buried assumptions, and beliefs as one technique to stimulate critical reflection and thinking.

ATTITUDES, TRAITS, AND SKILLS NEEDED FOR CRITICAL THINKING

Several authors suggest that there are both affective and cognitive aspects to thinking critically (Ennis, 1985; Norris & Ennis, 1989; Paul, 1990; Perry, 1970). They often define these as the affective attitudes and the cognitive skills of critical thinking. Green (2000) summarizes the affective attitudes and cognitive skills as follows.

Affective Attitudes of Critical Thinking:

- Intellectual humility—knowing/accepting limits of knowledge
- Intellectual courage—listen and fairly evaluate divergent views/ideas
- Intellectual empathy—imagine self in place of other
- Intellectual integrity—hold self to universal standard of proof
- Intellectual perseverance—search for truth worth the effort
- Faith in reason—best interests of humanity to develop thinking skills
- Intellectual sense of justice—assess all viewpoints without vested interest

Cognitive Skills of Critical Thinking

- Divergent thinking—analyze a diversity of opinions to determine relevancy
- Reasoning—inductive and deductive, general principles of logic
- Reflection—ponder, contemplate, deliberate (takes time)
- Creativity—produce ideas and alternatives, consider multiple solutions
- Clarification—note similarities and differences, define terms, assumptions
- Basic support—use of known facts and background knowledge

Hunter and Lops (1994) describe a Critical Thinking Process model adapted from Paul (1990) that includes standards, ability to reason, modes of reasoning, and traits of the mind surrounding elements of thought. Their list of traits of the mind adds intellectual curiosity, civility, responsibility, and discipline to the affective list summarized by Green, along with "developing insight into egocentricity or sociocentricity" (p. 45). This latter category is illumined through the critical reflection process described earlier, and allows for discussion of varying values and attitudes that are such an important part of being human (the reader is referred back to chapter 4 for a full discussion of values).

LIMITATIONS OF CRITICAL THINKING

The most important limitation of critical thinking is a personal unwillingness to think and to reflect on that thinking before taking action. This personal limitation is totally under the control of the individual learner, creating a high level of frustration for the teacher. Sometimes the learner does not realize why they are unwilling to spend the time and effort needed to think critically about a clinical situation and the decisions needed. At other times this unwillingness to think critically is the result of apathy, a lack of commitment to and/or interest in thinking, or a mistaken belief that one knows what the proper decision already is without any further thought—too often based on past experience without recognition that the current situation may be quite different than one's experience base. Likewise, lack of insight and limited understanding of one's values and biases detract from critical thinking and good decision-making.

Another limitation of critical thinking results from emergency situations where time is extremely limited and the clinician is required to act with a minimum of thought. It is in these emergency situations that the experienced clinician (the teacher) will depend on expert "knowing" as described by Benner (1984). Novice clinicians have minimal experience on which to base their quick analysis of an emergency situation, and may, in fact, need the teacher to take over or go into a "directing mode" of teaching—telling the learner what to do (Blanchard, 1985; Schon, 1993). Such a "telling" situation can become a positive learning experience provided that the teacher reviews the approach to the emergency in a post-conference after the situation is stabilized. Offering the learner the opportunity to "take over" in the next emergency is an important step in learning how to act in such situations with reassurance that the teacher will be present to support the learner.

Though emergency situations cannot be planned for nor really controlled, and it is often difficult to encourage a learner to think critically if they are not willing to do so, most other limitations of critical thinking can be overcome by teaching methods and teacher behaviors.

TEACHING METHODS

The challenge to the teacher of adults is to evaluate both the willingness of learners to think critically and their ability to do so (Facione & Facione, 1996a; Facione, Facione, & Sanchez, 1994). Creating the conditions for critical thinking is an essential step in fostering such thinking among others. There have been several studies of different teaching methodologies and their impact on learner's level of critical thinking, but with varying results as will be discussed below. Videbeck (1997) reported that the most common tool for measuring critical thinking used in nursing settings is the Watson Glaser Critical Thinking Appraisal (WGCTA) (Watson & Glaser, 1980). However, some results of using this standardized instrument at the beginning and end of a nursing student's educational program seem to indicate that learners who score low on critical thinking skills at the beginning of their educational program show a significant improvement at the end, and those who begin their nursing education with high critical thinking scores tend to score lower at the end of their program. Several explanations have been offered to explain this phenomenon, including senior students' lack of interest in completing the tool, the possible inappropriateness of using such a tool for measurement of thinking, or use of a curriculum that is not be designed to enhance critical thinking (Magnussen, Ishida, & Itano, 2000; McMillan, 1987; Vaughan-Wrobel, O'Sullivan, & Smith, 1997). Critical thinking may actually be suppressed by both a curriculum and teacher that require the learner to do it "one way" or "my way"—the teacher's way.

One of the more worrisome explanations for lack of change in or diminished ability to think critically among learners is that the dominant teaching methods used during nursing education actually curtail the development of critical thinking in those who are somewhat proficient in this process to begin with. In other words, as a teacher it is possible to turn off the inquisitive, reflective impulses in learners by the way we teach. It is, therefore, the responsibility of the teacher to create an environment of discovery, of thinking, of risk taking, of trust, and of acceptance that not all efforts to think will result in good actions or behaviors. Below is a brief discussion of teaching methods that can contribute to critical thinking in others.

Guided Imagery

One of the affective dimensions of critical thinking is self-reflection. Guided imagery has been used to promote such reflection as a part of challenging and then understanding the unknown, unconscious assumptions about people or ideas or concepts that all of us carry in our minds. These unconscious views can and do influence one's perception of a situation. If one is not willing to take the time to examine the "unknown" assumptions, one's ability to discover the variety of meaning and understanding in the situation will result in less than optimal interaction (relationships) with others and less than optimal decision-making.

Krejci (1997) describes the use of guided imagery in fostering critical thinking and reflection. She notes that one must engage the learner and seek permission to use this technique as it can be threatening to those who have not participated in such activity before. It is important to emphasize that learners do not have to participate, do not have to share their images with others, but are encouraged to do so. Setting a positive tone and having a comfortable and safe environment for imaging are also important steps. The learner is encouraged to take a comfortable position in their chair, to relax their body, and to close their eyes. Some teachers begin with slow, deep breathing and calming words to clear the learner's mind of the day's distractions/concerns. Then a selected word or concept (such as power, leadership, patient, nurse) is spoken by the teacher and the learners are asked to visualize this concept on the back of their closed eyelids. After a short time, the learners are asked to remember their images, take a deep breath, and slowly open their eyes. Each participant is asked to share their images while encouraging active listening in others. Judgments about images are not allowed whereas searching for meaning of such images is encouraged.

Guided imagery can be effectively used in beginning discussions of what it means to think critically and to illustrate the affective dimensions or traits of critical thinking. This method can also be used periodically throughout the graduate education program as new dimensions of the advanced practice role or new patient care situations demand an expanded view or understanding of thinking and action.

Case Studies

Case studies, whether prepared by the teacher-clinician or taken from learners' actual clinical experiences, are a time-honored tradition in health professions education. Case studies used as preparation for the first clinical rotation, as examination/discussion of ongoing clinical practice, or as part of the formative evaluation of learning can afford great opportunities for thinking, for problem solving, and for learning from others' experience in the safety of the classroom. The teacher needs to be aware that simply offering case studies for analysis and discussion does not guarantee that the learner will be guided to think critically. The way the case is structured, the approach to thinking about the situation includes encouraging alternative or "lateral" out-of-the-box thinking, and supporting learner efforts to go beyond the obvious to search for the unexpected, the unknown, or other meaning in the situation.

Case study analysis has often been equated with problem-based learning as originated at the McMaster University School of Medicine in the late 1960s. Several authors describe the components or process of problem-based learning as using clinical cases as an opportunity to use prior knowledge (from readings, class discussion, clinical experience) as a basis for understanding and organizing new information so that it can be transferred to new clinical situations. Key tools of problem-based learning include discussion, asking and answering questions, peer teaching, and critique. Albanese and Mitchell (1993) noted that problem-based learning as a teaching method focuses on the development of learner problem solving skills and for reinforcing basic knowledge needed to carry out the clinical role and responsibilities. This method, however, does not necessarily require critical thinking affective traits, and thus may not be the best choice of teaching methods for critical thinking (very useful for analysis of clinical practice, peer review, and quality improvement of practice through effective problem solving).

Inquiry-based learning was developed at the University of Hawaii at Manoa School of Nursing (UHSON) to add flexibility to problem-based learning. The faculty also included systems theory and collaboration (disciplinary as well as interdisciplinary) as integral components (Feletti, 1993). Inquiry based learning was defined as: "an orientation toward learning that is flexible and open, and draws on the varied skills and resources of faculty and students, in which faculty are co-learners who guide and facilitate the student-driven learning experience to achieve goals of nursing practice" (UHSON, 1992, p. 1). Magnussen, Ishida, and Itano (2000) used the Watson Glaser Critical Thinking Appraisal (WGCTA) to test whether inquiry-based learning would enhance critical thinking in learners. As in other studies of levels of critical thinking as measured by the WGCTA, students with the lowest scores at the beginning of their program gained significantly by the end of the program. This and other studies suggest that critical thinking can be taught, can be learned, and is most effective when working with those individuals who come to the health professions with limited abilities to think critically.

Some of the important points to consider as a teacher when using the case study method, especially when teaching critical thinking, are the need to 1) establish or select the cases to be used based on what the expected outcomes of learning are; 2) be present and facilitative (supporting, coaching) but not controlling (overly directive) during the discussions; and 3) be ready to correct misinformation or suggestions of unsafe practice, by either seeking from the group or offering the reasoning behind these corrections (depending on level of learner as new learners may not have the knowledge base to recognize errors in judgment).

Written Assignments

Written assignments can be used to examine the thinking ability of learners. Asking the learner to keep a log of self-reflection on the role of the advanced practice nurse or midwife is one activity that some learners enjoy. It is important for the teacher to clearly specify what should be written about in the log, and to read and offer feedback at pre-determined intervals. These logs often afford great opportunities for teacher-learner dialogue about the profession, about the growth from novice to advanced practitioner (Benner, 1984), and about the value of reflection on self-growth.

Another written assignment that is used to examine problem solving and critical analysis of evolving learner practice uses case studies that go beyond the traditional nursing care plan to problem solving. These written case analyses require clinical judgment with explanation of rationale or reasons for each decision made, and require alternative plans of action to meet the patient needs in the situation.

Socratic Questioning in the Clinical Area

One of the time-honored teaching techniques that fosters thinking, reflection, risk-taking, and decision-making in others is known as Socratic questioning. This type of questioning can be particularly effective in clinical teaching as the expert clinician-teacher asks the learner such things as, "What do you think might be going on in this situation?" or "What would you like to do?" or "What is your reason for selecting that particular treatment option for this patient?" or "Can you think of any other possible treatment or approach to this situation?" Any number of carefully worded questions can direct and support the learner to use existing knowledge and experience and apply it to the patient care situation at hand. If the teacher constantly gives the "correct" response without encouraging the learner to think it through themselves, the learner can develop a less than productive habit of the mind of memorizing the teacher's responses and then using them without further examination or thought. Not knowing why you have chosen to do or say or choose something can be disastrous in planning for individualized nursing or midwifery care. However, the teacher needs to understand that many novice learners can become easily frustrated when the teacher does not give the "answer" right away. The teacher needs to accept this frustration and know that in the long term having the learner think it through themselves will result in more internalization of learning and better patient care.

CRITERIA FOR MAKING GOOD DECISIONS

In a clinical practice discipline, it is important to know how to make decisions for and with others. Thinking about thinking is an important first step in being able to sort information, determine its relevance to decisions needed, and then proceed to analysis and supportive reasons for any final choice of action. This background on critical thinking leads to understanding the how and what of good decision-making in clinical practice. This chapter ends with a brief synopsis of the criteria for making good decisions in clinical practice and suggested ways to engage the learner in making such decisions.

It is often a helpful exercise with adult learners to ask them to think about a really good decision they have made recently in their lives as well as a decision they would classify as less than good. After a brief time for thought and reflection, the teacher can then proceed directly to ask the following questions: 1) What are the personal attributes that contribute to one's ability to make good decisions in one's daily life? 2) What knowledge is essential to making good decisions? and 3) What environmental conditions foster good decision-making? Many of the responses will often come directly from the adult learner who is drawing upon their own personal and extensive life experiences when they made good decisions as well as those times when they made a bad decision. Assisting the learner to reflect upon and analyze the elements of decision-making in both situations is yet another opportunity to reinforce the concept of critical thinking.

Personal Attributes

The list of personal attributes of particular importance in a clinical discipline include a healthy dose of common sense, humility, human sensitivity, and a pervasive calmness (at least outwardly). Personal values that respect self and others and understand what it means to be accountable for the outcomes of one's decisions are seen as basic to one's ability to think before acting, to admit errors in judgment, and to have the courage to make another decision or choice if needed. The willingness to make decisions along with the capacity to think critically (commitment to critical thinking) are also essential attributes for good decision-making. Here it may be important to emphasize with the learner that there are risks that go along with a willingness to think critically and make decisions in clinical practice. These risks include the time it takes to think and decide, the emotional investment in understanding self and others in the situation, the willingness to listen to alternative approaches to the situation (especially when they differ from one's own reasoned perspective), and the fact that sometimes the decision one makes is very unpopular, with all the resultant emotions.

Essential Knowledge

Enlightened knowledge of self (values, attitudes, biases) contributes to good decision-making, especially when a clinician is called upon to make decisions in practice with and for others. Access to pertinent information about the patient, the situation, limitations and/or constraints, coupled with a clear understanding of the particular health or illness condition that requires attention are other important areas of knowledge needed for making good decisions. Professional knowledge including illuminating and useful ethical principles that can be used to support one's choice of action leads to optimal decision-making as well. It is vital for the learner to understand professional knowledge at the level which it can be applied to the care of patients. This understanding includes knowing how to reason, to weigh options, to balance interests, and to finally select a path of action with or without discussion with other trusted colleagues. Knowing what you know and what you do not know, and being willing to seek help when needed is one of the hallmarks of a good clinician—a good thinker—a good decision-maker.

Environmental Attributes

Some of the environmental conditions that contribute to good decision-making in a clinical discipline include time, mutual trust based on respect for one another that leads to sharing of goals and preferences, and a commitment to maintaining the confidentiality of patient information to the extent possible. A supportive environment for learning an advanced practice role must allow for mistakes in reasoning and judgment, must clearly delineate the boundaries of safety for the novice clinician and protect him/her from harming others while learning. Practicing making decisions in clinical practice is a must, and many opportunities to practice this skill are required during the educational program. Reinforcement of sound reasoning as it occurs can turn tentative decision-making into confident decision-making—the goal of any professional practitioner.

SUMMARY

Critical thinking is vital to any health professional's practice. Critical thinking can be learned and it can be taught. Setting the environment for thinking, requiring thinking at all times, modeling critical thinking, and selecting teaching methods that enhance the learner's ability to think critically are the primary responsibilities of the teacher—whether in the classroom, on the computer, or in the clinical area.

REFLECTIONS

When you stop to think about thinking, what comes to mind? Have you ever thought about how you could teach others to think in an orderly, critical manner? How would you do it? What are some of the teaching methods you are currently using that support critical thinking in learners? Which would you change and why? Reflect on why an emphasis on thinking is needed for advanced practice nursing and midwifery practice.

SUGGESTED CLASSROOM EXERCISES

1. Select one or two images that require thoughtful consideration of less than obvious characteristics, such as the classic picture that includes the image of the old woman and young woman. Ask for first impressions from the group (the obvious), then ask if anyone sees something different.

2. Facilitate guided imaging of an advanced practice nurse or of a midwife. Follow with sharing and discussion of images and help learners identify those

perceptions (views) of these health professionals that are true today and those that are not, with reasons for why they are not today's reality.

REFERENCES

Albanese, M. A., & Mitchell, S. (1993). Problem-based learning: A review of literature on its outcomes and implementation issues. *Academic Medicine, 68*(1), 52–81.

Alfaro-LeFevre, R. (1995). *Critical thinking in nursing: A practical approach.* Philadelphia: W. B. Saunders.

Baker, C. R. (1996). Reflective learning: A teaching strategy for critical thinking. *Journal of Nursing Education, 35*(1), 19–22.

Bandman, E., & Bandman, B. (1995). *Critical thinking in nursing,* 2nd edition. Norwalk, CT: Appleton and Lange.

Belenky, M. F., Clinchy, B. M., Goldberger, N. R., & Tarule, J. M. (1986). Women's ways of knowing: The development of self, voice and mind. New York: Basic Books.

Benner, P. (1984). *From novice to expert: Excellence and power in clinical nursing practice.* Menlo Park: Addison Wesley.

Blanchard, K. (1985). *Situational leadership II.* Escondido, CA: Blanchard Training and Development Corporation.

Brookfield, S. D. (1987). *Developing critical thinkers: Challenging adults to explore alternative ways of thinking and acting.* Milton Keynes: Open University Press.

Cascio, R. S., Campbell, S., Sandor, M. K., Rains, A. P., & Clark, M. C. (1995). Enhancing critical thinking skills. *Nurse Educator, 20*(2), 38–43.

Daloz, L. A. (1986). *Effective teaching and mentoring.* San Francisco: Jossey-Bass.

Daly, W. M. (1998). Critical thinking as an outcome of nursing education. What is it? Why is it important to nursing practice? *Journal of Advanced Nursing, 28*(2), 323–331.

Dobrzykowski, T. M. (1994). Teaching strategies to promote critical thinking skills in nursing staff. *The Journal of Continuing Education in Nursing, 25*(6), 272–276.

Ennis, R. (1985). *A taxonomy of critical thinking dispositions and abilities.* Champaign, IL: University of Illinois Critical Thinking Project.

Facione, N. C., Facione, P. A., & Sanchez, C. A. (1994). Critical thinking disposition as a measure of competent clinical judgement: The development of the California Critical Thinking Disposition Inventory. *Journal of Nursing Education, 33*(8), 345–350.

Facione, N. C., & Facione, P. A. (1996a). Assessment design issues for evaluation critical thinking in nursing. *Holistic Nursing Practice, 10*(3), 41–53.

Facione, N. C., & Facione, P. A. (1996b). Externalizing the critical thinking in knowledge development and clinical judgement. *Nursing Outlook, 44*(3), 129–136.

Faciones, P. A. (1990). *The California Critical Thinking Skills Test (CCTST): Form A.* Millbrae, CA: California Academic Press.

Feletti, G. (1993). Inquiry-based and problem-based learning: How similar are these approaches to nursing and medical education? *Higher Education Research & Development, 12*(2), 143–156.

Ford, J. S., & Profetto-McGrath, J. (1994). A model of critical thinking within the context of curriculum as praxis. *Journal of Nursing Education, 33*(8), 341–344.

Freire, P. (1972). *Pedagogy of the oppressed.* Harmondworth, UK: Penguin.

Gordon, J. M. (2000). Congruency in defining critical thinking by nurse educators and non-nurse scholars. *Journal of Nursing Education, 39*(8), 340–351.

Green, C. (2000). *Critical thinking in nursing: Case studies across the curriculum.* Upper Saddle River, NJ: Prentice Hall Health.

Harbison, J. (1991). Clinical decision making in nursing. *Journal of Advanced Nursing, 16,* 404–407.

Henderson, V. (1982). Nursing process—is the title right? *Journal Advanced Nursing, 7,* 103–109.

Hunter, L. P., & Lops, V. R. (1994). Critical thinking and the nurse-midwifery management process. *Journal of Nurse-Midwifery, 39*(1), 43–46.

Jones, A., & Brown, L. N. (1991). Critical thinking: Impact on nursing education. *Journal of Advanced Nursing, 16,* 529–533.

Kataoka-Yahiro, M., & Saylor, C. (1994). A critical thinking model for nursing judgement. *Journal of Nursing Education, 33*(8), 351–356.

Knowles, M. S., & Associates. (1984). *Andragogy in action: Applying modern principles of adult learning.* San Francisco: Jossey-Bass.

Krejci, J. W. (1997). Imagery: Stimulating critical thinking by exploring mental models. *Journal of Nursing Education, 36*(10), 482–484.

Magnussen, L., Ishida, D., & Itano, J. (2000). The impact of the use of inquiry-based learning as a teaching methodology on the development of critical thinking. *Journal of Nursing Education, 39*(8), 360–364.

McMillan, J. (1987). Enhancing college students' critical thinking: A review of studies. *Research in Higher Education, 26*(1), 3–29.

Mezirow, J. (1991). *Transformative dimensions of adult learning.* San Francisco: Jossey-Bass.

Norris, S. P. (1985). Synthesis of research on critical thinking. *Educational Leadership, 42*(8), 40–45.

Norris, S. P., & Ennis, R. (1989). *Evaluating critical thinking.* Pacific Grove, CA: Critical Thinking Press and Software.

Oermann, M. H. (1998). How to assess critical thinking in clinical practice. *Dimensions of Critical Care Nursing, 17*(6), 322–327.

Paul, R. (1990). *Critical thinking.* Rohnert Park, CA: The Center for Critical Thinking and Moral Critique, Sonoma State University.

Paul, R., & Heaslip, P. (1995). Critical thinking and intuitive nursing practice. *Journal of Advanced Nursing, 22,* 40–70.

Perry, W. (1970). *Forms of intellectual and ethical development in the college years: The scheme.* New York: Holt, Rinehart & Winston.

Phillips, D. A. (2000). Language as constitutive: Critical thinking for multicultural education and practice in the 21st century. *Journal of Nursing Education, 39*(8), 365–372.

Rubenfeld, M. G., & Scheffer, B. K. (1995). *Critical thinking in nursing: An interactive approach.* Philadelphia: J. B. Lippincott.

Scheffer, B. K., & Rubenfeld, M. G. (2000). A consensus statement on critical thinking in nursing. *Journal of Nursing Education, 39*(8), 352–359.

Schon, D. A. (1983). *The reflective practitioner: How professionals think in action.* New York: Basic Books.

Shor, I., & Freire, P. (1987). *A pedagogy for liberation: Dialogues on transforming education*. Grandby, MA: Bergin and Garvin.

Tanner, C. A. (1996). Critical thinking revisited: Paradoxes and emerging perspectives. *Journal of Nursing Education, 35*(1), 3–4.

Tanner, C. A. (1999). Evidence-based practice: Research and critical thinking. *Journal of Nursing Education, 38*(3), 99.

Tanner, C. A. (2000). Critical thinking: Beyond nursing process. *Journal of Nursing Education, 39*(8), 338–339.

University of Hawaii School of Nursing. (1992). *Faculty statement*. Honolulu: Author.

Vaughn-Wrobel, B. C., O'Sullivan, P., & Smith, L. (1997). Evaluating critical thinking skills of baccalaureate nursing students. *Journal of Nursing Education, 36*(10), 485–488.

Videbeck, S. L. (1997). Critical thinking: Prevailing practice in baccalaureate schools of nursing. *Journal of Nursing Education, 36*(1), 5–10.

Watson, G., & Glaser, E. M. (1980). *Watson-Glaser Critical Thinking Appraisal, Forms A and B*. New York: Psychological Corporation.

White, N., Beardslee, N., Peters, D., & Supples, J. (1990). Promoting critical thinking skills. *Nurse Educator, 15*(5), 16–19.

CHAPTER 6

The Influence of Age, Race/ Ethnicity, Culture, and Gender

There are no bad students only discouraged ones.

—Anonymous

SUGGESTED OUTCOMES FOR THIS CHAPTER

At the completion of this chapter the reader will be able to

1. compare and contrast developmental theories that view the significant aspects of development as sequential patterns (stage theories), or as life events (transitions theories), and
2. describe how sociocultural factors influence teaching and learning.

INTRODUCTION

A number of factors influence the educational experience of individuals and groups. In the past consideration of individual physical and psychological changes was deemed sufficient in the study of learner variables affecting the learning experience. More recently, educators, faced with an increasingly diverse student body, have realized the importance of race/ethnicity, gender, socioeconomics, and culture on the learning experience. Recent studies address these issues, but the body of knowledge we currently have may be inadequate to address these factors in their entirety. An ongoing awareness of the influence of these factors is essential for today's educators.

PHYSICAL CHANGES IN ADULTHOOD

We continue to see a wide diversity in the ages of our learners. Some are newly graduated from BSN programs and between the ages of 21 and 25, some are nurses with a few years of clinical experience and may be in their late 20s to mid to late 30s. Those who fall within these ages are stable in their physical development and if they have no physical illness typically experience no physical impediment to continuing their education. We also have a cadre of learners whose ages range from early 40s to mid to early 60s. These learners are the ones most likely to experience some of the physical changes associated with midlife.

Changes in the Senses

Visual changes may be the most noticeable ones that individuals experience in midlife. Presbyopia almost universally affects midlife adults' ability to focus for near vision. Those who have never worn glasses find themselves relying more and more on corrective glasses in order to read. In classes that use both print and projected media the learner is frequently forced to shift fields of vision from distant to close and this can be a source of stress as the learner struggles to continually readjust his/her focus. Although easily corrected, presbyopia reminds the student that s/he is aging and that adjustments need to be made during this process. This may be a source of stress for some learners and certainly requires some readjustment of the learner's self-image.

Auditory changes, although they may be less frequent than visual changes, can be more difficult to manage. Because these changes are often subtle they may go undetected and therefore uncorrected. Often, instruction is based on auditory methods. Awareness of the possibility of the middle/older aged learners' auditory difficulty can help with early detection and correction.

Changes in Overall Health

Overall health may decrease as age increases. The incidence of chronic illness and the use of a variety of medications increase with age and can influence the learner's ability to be successful. Fatigue is often a sequellae of chronic illness and can interfere with the learner's ability to concentrate, endure long teaching sessions, and attend class. Medication can also affect the learner's ability to concentrate, solve problems, and attend to the task at hand. Concerns about health can also divert the learner's ability to focus on the educational process.

PSYCHOLOGICAL DEVELOPMENT IN ADULTHOOD

Theories concerning psychological development have long been divided into two types, sequential or stage/phase theories, and life event or transition theories. Current approaches to adult psychological development consider the influence of gender, race, culture, and contextual and environmental factors in the development process. We will first consider the classic theories of psychological development and then move on to the newer more inclusive approaches to adult psychological development.

Sequential or Stage/Phase Theories

Generally, stage/phase theories posit that development occurs in a series of stages that are related to age or a specific period in one's life. Individuals move from simple to complex thinking about self and work. Life tasks make for learning readiness and create "teachable moments" (Merriam & Caffarella, 1991). Erickson is perhaps one of the most prominent stage/phase theorists. Many are familiar with his eight stages of development that are hierarchical in nature and depend on the sequential completion of the tasks for each stage (Erickson, 1959). Three tasks are central to the adult phases of his theory. In early adulthood the task is intimacy, in the second stage of adulthood the task is generativity, and the final task is integrity. The first task is accomplished through establishing one or more intimate relationships. The next task is accomplished through redirecting attention from self to others and supporting the next generation. The final task is accomplished through "the acceptance of one's one and only life cycle and the people who have become significant to it as something that had to be and that, by necessity, permitted no substitutions" (Erickson, 1959, p. 139).

Another well-known stage theorist, Levinson, sees development during the adult years as progressing through orderly steps that are dependent upon age. He sees development as a series of stable times interspersed with times of transition, with the focus of life on the boundary between self and other (Levinson, 1986). Each period of time has developmental tasks. These tasks revolve around an individual's relationships with others—individuals and groups, institutions, and cultures. These alternating periods of stability and transition are divided into four eras. Three of the eras occur in adulthood. Early adulthood, age 17–45, is characterized by the greatest demands from family, community, and society.

Middle adulthood, ages 40–65, is characterized by an energetic, socially valuable, and personally satisfying existence. The individual has not only accomplished their own work but is also involved in the development of the current generation of young adults. Older adulthood, age 65 and over, is a time when the individual confronts the self and makes peace with the world (Levinson, 1986).

Both of these theorists base their theories on research done with white, middle class American males as subjects. Recently, researchers in the field have called into question some of the assumptions of both theorists and their applicability to individuals of different races, ethnicities, and gender, as well as individuals living within a different sociopolitical era.

Life Events and Transitions Theories

Those with a life events/transitions approach to development ascribe to the centrality of social or life events and how they stimulate transitions and consequently development. These theorists recognize individual variability in human behavior and do not believe, like stage theorists, that human behavior is more or less universal, biologically driven, and perhaps age related. There are two basic types of life events, individual and cultural. Individual life events are events such as birth, serious illness, and divorce. Examples of cultural life events are wars and the women's movement (Merriam & Caffarella, 1991).

Schlossberg (1988), a well-known transitions theorist, considers transitions as events or nonevents that alter adult lives. Some examples of these are the birth of a child, marriage or not marrying, divorce, job loss, and retirement. The more these events alter an individual's role in life the greater the effect of the transition. These transitions, rather than chronological age, affect an individual's understanding and evaluation of human behavior. Transitions are viewed as opportunities for individuals to reevaluate and reexamine their life course. They serve as triggers that stimulate adults to grow and learn. How individuals cope with these transitions depends on the balance between their strengths/resources and the deficits in their lives. Although individuals cannot control the timing or intensity of these transitions they can affect the outcome by how they utilize their strengths and resources and they can become more skilled in dealing with transitions over time.

Bridges (1991), another transitions theorist, defines transition as a "psychological process people go through" (p. 3). This process allows them to cope with a disorienting event. He believes there are three phases in each transition: ending, neutral zone, and new beginning. Ending or letting go of the past allows the individual to start the process of transition. Neutral zone occurs after letting go and when the individual extinguishes old non-adaptive behaviors and begins the development of new patterns of behaviors to cope with the change. The final phase, the new beginning, happens when coping behaviors are established and life goes on.

As in stage/phase theories, research on transition theory of adult development has focused on white, American, middle class males, and suffers from the same criticism as stage/phase theories research.

NEWER THEORIES OF ADULT DEVELOPMENT

More recent work on adult psychological development is concerned with the effect of gender, race/ethnicity, culture, and socioeconomics on the development of adults. Building on the previous work of developmental theorists, these new theorists have studied women, African Americans, Native Americans, Asian Americans, and individuals from a variety of social classes. The effects of gender, ethnicity/race, and socioeconomics are key to their theories.

Adult Development and Gender

As noted above, in the past developmental theorists conducted their studies on white, middle class, American males, and then generalized their findings to include women and other groups. Starting in the 1980s a number of researchers began to explore the possibility that gender affects adult development and that perhaps the findings of male adult development were not totally generalizable to women (Ross-Gordon, 1999).

Two of the early researchers in gender and development were Gilligan (1982) and Josselson (1987). Gilligan reexamined Kohlberg's work on moral development and studied women's ethical decision-making. She found that women base their moral decision-making on an ethic of caring, while men base their moral decision-making on an ethic of justice. Josselson (1987) reexamined Erickson's work and found that being able to maintain a sense of connectedness, which was never considered in Erickson's work with men, was essential in women's development.

Caffarella and Olson (1993) reviewed the literature on women's psychological development and noted the central importance of connection over separation in women's lives. This is in opposition to the previous view, based on male dominated studies, that autonomy is central to adult development. They also noted that women have diverse and nonlinear patterns of development.

It is clear that gender strongly influences adult development. There are differences between the way men and women experience adult development. There is, however, never one absolute way in which individuals behave/develop. It is important to note that other influences such as race/ethnicity also affect adult development, and universal statements concerning the way all women or all men experience development will prove to be inadequate.

Race/Ethnicity and Adult Development

As the population of the United States has become more diverse it has become apparent that it is necessary to consider the effects of race/ethnicity on many aspects of our culture. Demographic data indicate that the population is changing from a predominantly European white population to one made up of groups previously thought of as minorities—African Americans, Hispanic Americans, and Asian Americans (Guy, 1999).

For centuries, white Americans have made up the mainstream of American society. "For them, ethnicity is usually invisible and unconscious because societal norms have been constructed around their racial, ethnic, and cultural frameworks, values and priorities and then referred to as 'standard American culture' rather than as 'ethnic identity' " (Chavez & Guido-DiBrito, 1999, p. 39). The shift in American demographics has begun to challenge this unconscious Eurocentric culture and its norms.

As a result of their race/ethnicity, learners bring different sets of expectations to the learning experience. These expectations are based on previous learning experiences, and interactions with teachers and peers. Members of the nondominant ethnic groups have had to adjust during their learning experiences to the norms and values of the dominant group. Some have been more successful than others in this adjustment. Now, we are striving to provide a more culturally appropriate learning experience for students so that success can be available to all.

The most important activity for educators concerning race/ethnicity is to develop an awareness of our own racially and ethnically defined sense of self, beliefs about learning, and education. We need to examine what we believe about members of an ethnic group that is different than ours. Negative beliefs and stereotypes are learned through cultural institutions and practices. Learning about our own culture/ethnicity and other groups occurs in childhood through socialization by parents, media, and peers. Often these beliefs and stereotypes remain unexamined and in some cases unconscious. Unexamined, they will certainly influence our behavior.

In addition to understanding our own beliefs, an understanding of the cultural norms of a variety of learners is imperative if the learning environment is to be inclusive. It is important to balance different cultural norms in considering the types of learning activities and assignments, as well as expectations about class participation. Without this consideration, the environment in which education takes places is unconsciously culturally constructed in line with the culture of the teacher.

Integrating discussion of the effects of race/ethnicity and culture on learning, health, and health care in the curriculum allows for learners to begin to become aware of the importance of identifying their own feelings on race/ethnicity. The teacher's role is to maintain a nonjudgmental atmosphere and facilitate a sense of respect for multiple perspectives.

As our learner population becomes increasingly diverse we, as educators, will be concerned about the effects of age, race/ethnicity, culture, and gender on the learner and the learning climate. It is necessary to develop an openness and concern about these areas and keep abreast of the latest research. Nothing, however, substitutes for simply talking with individuals about their perceptions of the learning experience, their interpretation of how these factors affect their learning and interactions with peers, and what they perceive would be helpful in their educational experience. Even though we have information about general characteristics of specific groups we can never lose sight of the individual. All the individuals in a specific group may not share the same characteristics.

REFLECTIONS

Think about your experiences with individuals from different ethnic or cultural backgrounds. What were some of the stereotypes you had heard over the years about this particular group of people? Did you feel that the stereotypes were accurate? Was your expectation that these individuals should adjust to your ethnic/cultural values and beliefs?

REFERENCES

Bridges, W. (1991). *Managing transitions: Making the most of change.* Reading, MA: Addison Wessley.

Caffarella, R., & Olson, S. K. (1993). Psychosocial development of women: A critical review of the literature. *Adult Education Quarterly, 43*(3), 125–151.

Chavez, A. F., & Guido-DiBrito, F. (1999). Racial and ethnic identity and development. *New Directions for Adult and Continuing Education, 84,* 39–47.

Erickson, E. H. (1959). *Identity and the life cycle.* New York: Norton.

Gilligan, C. (1981). *In a different voice: Psychological theory and women's development.* Cambridge, MA: Harvard University Press.

Guy, T. (1999). Culture as context for adult education: The need for culturally relevant adult education. *New Directions for Adult and Continuing Education, 82,* 7–17.

Josselson, R. (1987). *Finding herself: Pathways to identity development in women.* San Francisco: Jossey-Bass.

Levinson, D. J. (1986). A conception of adult development. *American Psychologist, 41*(1), 3–13.

Merriam, S., & Caffarella, R. (1991). *Learning in adulthood.* San Francisco: Jossey-Bass.

Ross-Gordon, J. M. (1999). Gender development and gendered adult development. *New Directions for Adult and Continuing Education, 84,* 29–36.

Schlossberg, N. (1988). Managing adult transitions. *Training and Development Journal, 42*(12), 58–60.

CHAPTER 7

Curriculum Development

> The development of a curriculum not only requires a commitment to the conviction that the learning opportunities we offer are in the best interest of the student, the profession, and society, but also demands the courage to make appropriate changes when these learning experiences are no longer useful to the goals of the curriculum.
> —Virginia C. Conley,
> *Curriculum and Instruction in Nursing*

SUGGESTED OUTCOMES FOR THIS CHAPTER

At the completion of this chapter and selected readings, the reader should

1. have insight into the historical evolution of the curriculum process in nursing,
2. be able to define the components essential to curriculum development, and
3. be able to describe the curriculum development process.

HISTORICAL PERSPECTIVE

Advanced practice nursing is the result of a natural progression in the development of nursing education and practice. In order to understand the curriculum process, which directs the implementation of advanced practice nursing and midwifery, it is useful to briefly review curriculum development in a historical perspective. It is beyond the scope of this book to do a detailed survey of the history of nursing and midwifery beyond the content in chapter 1, but in order to understand curriculum development in the new millennium, a brief overview is presented.

Nursing has always been one of the innovative disciplines in the health care arena. As early as 1893, 40 superintendents of training schools had agreed to form an organization, the Society of Superintendents, to establish and maintain a universal standard of training. This organization was renamed the National League for Nursing Education and eventually the National League for Nursing. In 1917 a milestone was reached with the publication of the *Standard Curriculum for Schools of Nursing*. With this publication, nursing reached a new level of refinement in its efforts to establish an improved and more standard curriculum across the country (Murdock, 1983). Revisions in the document were made in 1927 and 1937. The title was changed to *A Curriculum Guide for Schools of Nursing* in the 1937 publication. In 1950 the National League for Nursing Education placed curriculum development under the direction of the faculty of each school based on standards developed by the profession.

Nursing continued to respond to emerging societal changes and specifically to the development of the study of curriculum as a specialized field within educational theory. A number of psychologists and educators from higher education, through their ongoing study and publications, contributed to the specific curricula developed by nursing faculty. Tyler's *Basic Principles of Curriculum and Instruction* (1949) served as the framework and underpinning of nursing curricula. Concepts emphasized by Tyler include instructional objectives; selection of learning experiences utilizing the criteria of continuity, sequence and integration; and evaluation based on instructional objectives. Taba (1962) further developed the original work of Tyler and in her work noted that there were only a few scattered remarks available in the curriculum literature about the functions of a curriculum theory or a conceptual framework in designing curriculum (p. 420). She did contribute to the elimination of this vacuum by devoting one chapter in her work to a conceptual framework. The publication of Bloom, Engelhart, Furst, Hill, and Krathwohl (1956) provided nurse educators with a clear taxonomy of behavioral objectives that contributed to the ongoing development of nursing curricula. These concepts were further developed by nurse educators in the context of nursing curricula, as evidenced in the work of Heidgerken (1953), Conley (1973), Bevis (1973), and Torres (1974), and became fundamental to curriculum design in schools and colleges of nursing.

DEVELOPMENT OF NURSING THEORY AND A CONCEPTUAL FRAMEWORK

A turning point in the discipline of nursing was the doctorate in nursing movement of the 1970s and 1980s that promoted the development of nursing knowledge.

Carper (1978), Donaldson and Crowley (1978), Chinn and Jacobs (1983), and Fawcett (1984) are examples of this new paradigm. One of the greatest contributions by the emerging nurse scholars was the subsequent development of conceptual frameworks that moved nursing education and practice from the medical model to a nursing model. Considerable agreement now exists that the central concepts of nursing are: person, environment, health, and nursing (Fawcett, 1989). A number of nurse scholars have developed nursing theories and conceptual models of nursing. Some of the conceptual models on which advanced nursing curricula and advanced nursing practice are based include Johnson's (1980) Behavioral Systems Model, King's (1981) Interacting Systems Framework, Levine's (1980) Conservation Model, Neuman's (1982) Systems Model, Orem's (1985) Self Care Framework, and Roy's (1984) Adaptation Model. The advanced practice nursing programs are beneficiaries of the new paradigm.

As indicated in the previous paragraphs the discipline of nursing is dynamic and responsive to societal changes and needs. The 1987 Fourth Nursing Education Conference "Curriculum Development Revolution" provided a forum for a critical assessment of nursing curricula and a call to "deinstitutionalize the Tyler curriculum model" (Bevis, 1988, p. 35). What had originated as a guide to curriculum development was now perceived as a code. The major criticism of the Tyler model is that "the Tyler model is based on behaviorist-learning theory, and behaviorism lends itself to training, not to education" (Bevis, 1988, p. 33). Recognition was given to the positive role of the Tyler model but also to the negative aspect of being "the only sanctioned model in nursing" (Bevis, 1988, p. 33).

The revolution was a response to a variety of issues and brought into focus new paradigms that are central to advanced practice nursing curriculum development. These paradigms, which have been presented in previous chapters, include critical thinking, student-teacher dialogue, human caring, feminist pedagogy, and adult learning theories.

NURSE-MIDWIFERY

Traditionally midwifery programs in the United States were developed as a certificate program for registered nurses or in master's degree programs for the graduate of a Bachelor of Science in a nursing program. The paradigm shifts which took place in nursing were less relevant for midwifery as by its very nature midwifery has always had a humanistic philosophy. The philosophy of care is characterized by caring, nurturing, and the recognition of the role of intuition in the care process. Critical thinking is an underlying principle in midwifery management process, and is central to midwifery care.

DETERMINING FACTORS OF CURRICULUM DEVELOPMENT

Bevis (1973) identified the theoretical framework as the curriculum keystone, which she defined as "the conceptualization and articulation of theories, phenomena, and variables relevant to a specific nursing educational system" (p. 19). She further defined the essential components in this framework as the structural and cognitive components.

The structural components basic to curriculum development include the educational setting, organization and purpose of the institution, and learner/teacher characteristics. For the development of advanced practice curricula in the new millennium, information related to the educational setting is available by accessing the criteria for the accreditation process of the specific advanced practice program and requirements for certification of the advanced practitioner. Guidelines of the National Organization of Nurse Practitioner Faculties are available for the advanced nursing programs, as well as criteria for schools of nurse midwifery/midwifery accredited by the American College of Nurse-Midwives, Division of Accreditation (DOA). Prior to initiating a new program a careful study should be undertaken of the organization and purpose of the parent institution in which the advanced practice nursing program will be placed, i.e. the philosophy of the parent institution, institutional support, and intra-professional support. Learner/teacher characteristics to be considered include the pool from which the learners will be selected, the professional qualifications and quality of the available lecturers and instructors, and the autonomy for the practice of the teachers and learners in order to attain the goals of the program. The cognitive components of the theoretical framework described by Bevis—philosophy, nursing theories, and learning theories—have been discussed in other chapters.

Advances in nursing knowledge have enabled nursing to move forward and more clearly articulate conceptual models of nursing and use this conceptual framework as the general outline for curriculum content and teaching/learning activities. "When a conceptual model is used for curriculum construction, it must be linked with theories about education and the teaching learning process, as well as with substantive theoretical content from nursing and adjunctive disciplines. The resulting conceptual-theoretical-empirical system then applies to the nursing participant, the student and the educator" (Fawcett, 2000, p. 41).

Fawcett (2000) has identified five rules inherent in each conceptual model relevant to the curricular structure and educational processes:

1. The first rule identifies the distinctive focus of the curriculum and the purposes to be fulfilled by nursing education.
2. The second rule identifies the general nature and sequence of the content to be presented.

3. The third rule identifies the settings in which nursing education occurs.
4. The fourth rule identifies the characteristics of legitimate students.
5. The fifth rule identifies the teaching learning strategies to be employed.

INTRODUCTION TO THE SPECIFICS OF CURRICULUM DEVELOPMENT

No attempt will be made to present an in-depth discussion of the curriculum process and curriculum development. This information is readily available in the educational and nursing literature (see Bevis, 1982; Bevis & Watson, 1989; McNeil, 1985; and Torres & Stanton, 1982). Rather, an overview focusing on the schema of the curriculum process will be presented as a reminder of the responsibility inherent in accepting the teacher role. The goal is to provide a foundation and familiarity with curricular concepts that can be used as building blocks for further study and application.

Conley (1973) defined curriculum as the content and processes of relationships between students, teachers, and others, and the arrangement of the physical and social environments that facilitate the attainment of specified goals that are consistent with and an integral part of the total school program. She elaborated further by stating that curriculum and instruction are inseparable and involve both interaction and transaction. It is interesting to note Conley's understanding of the teacher-student roles many years prior to the "curriculum revolution." Torres and Stanton (1982) state that the curriculum process involves a systematic approach to the development of organized learning and its related aspects. Bevis (1982) defines curriculum as the totality of learning activities that are designed to achieve specific educational outcomes. A changing perspective can be noted in Bevis (1989) with her definition of curriculum as "transactions and interactions that take place between and among students and teachers with the intent that learning takes place" (p. 72).

Two important concepts related to curriculum are—it is a process and it is systematic. The curriculum process is systematic, logical, dynamic, and spiraled in nature since it reflects all characteristics of a process (Torres & Stanton, 1982, p. 26). In order to grasp the process it is presented diagrammatically in Appendix A but it must be understood it is not a linear process.

The curriculum process is the means that enables the faculty, as a unified group, to articulate their philosophy (values and beliefs) about person, environment, health, and nursing as well as agreed statements related to adult teaching and learning and concepts such as human caring, critical thinking, student-teacher dialogue, and feminist pedagogy. The agreed philosophy must be a living philosophy and one that has faculty consensus and commitment. It should reflect the conceptual framework that will drive the curriculum and concepts that indicate the nurse or midwife is being prepared for an independent and collaborative role. A glossary of terms used in the philosophy is essential in order to ensure equal understanding of the terminology by the learners and educators using the curriculum.

The philosophy serves as the foundation for the characteristics of the graduates, the curriculum design, content, teaching methods and strategies, and student and program evaluation. Each advanced practice curriculum has a uniqueness based on the health care needs of the population it is designed to serve and the theoretical model it selects to meet these health care needs. A nursing or midwifery model is required if a nursing or midwifery perspective rather than a medical perspective is to be the foundation for the program.

The next issue to be addressed is the development and clarification of the conceptual theoretical framework building on the concepts and the relationships of these concepts already described in the philosophy. Torres (1974) recommends the use of vertical and horizontal strands to provide an integrated curriculum. She defines vertical strands as content threads identified in the theoretical framework that are used to identify and plan progressive learning experiences that build one upon the other throughout the nursing courses; and horizontal strands as process-oriented threads identified in the theoretical framework that are constantly used and reinforced throughout each nursing course in the curriculum. These strands, imbedded in the philosophy and conceptual framework, need identification and consensus in order to promote a unified whole. The conceptual framework will direct the stated outcomes of the program, the selection of content and learning experiences, and the evaluation process. For ease of understanding, the conceptual theoretical framework is diagrammed as a step but should not be interpreted as a linear process. It is reflected in all the phases of the curriculum.

Outcomes for the program or statements of outcome competencies are inclusive of knowledge, skills, behaviors, and values. For example, if human caring is a central concept in the philosophy of the program, this should be reflected in the outcomes. Outcomes are derived from position statements and curriculum guidelines issued from the various advanced practice nursing and midwifery organizations and expert nursing practice. Development of outcomes takes into consideration current research on nursing needs and roles in a changing health care system. The program outcome competencies encompass unit and course outcomes.

Progression through a program can be determined by units, levels, or other designated systems. Each of these intermediate designations has outcome competencies based on the didactic and clinical courses included in the designation. The focus of all outcome competencies is the learner.

Discrete outcome competencies are required for each course. The course outcome competencies include cognitive (knowledge), psychomotor (skills), and affective (values and behaviors) domains that are observable and can be appraised. It is at this level that critical decisions are made as to what content must be included to enable the learner to attain the desired competency and what can be excluded.

Learning activities, teaching methods, and strategies are identified as a means to enhance the teaching-learning outcomes. Principles of adult learning and interactive teaching methods have been discussed in previous chapters. Selection of teaching methods cannot be left to chance. Selection is based on the competency to be attained and individual and group learner needs.

Methods for appraisal of student performance and appraisal of program effectiveness, an integral part of curriculum development, are identified for formative and summative appraisal. Appraisal is reviewed in a later chapter.

Curriculum development is a learned process. It is a dynamic and very creative process. It is a response to advances in nursing knowledge and to the health care needs of society. Although developed to meet the needs as identified at the time of the initial development or revision, it must have sufficient flexibility to incorporate emerging evidence-based educational and clinical practice research. A curriculum should never be a static document. Ongoing course and program evaluation is the basis for curriculum revision.

Curriculum Design

Torres and Stanton (1982) define curriculum design as the organization and sequencing of course requirements and learning experiences that comprise the total program. All curriculum designs have essentially the same concerns: learners, subject matter, and educational processes (Conley, 1973). The 2001 Standards and Criteria Document of the National League for Nursing Accrediting Commission (NLNAC) addresses curriculum design as the responsibility of the faculty, "Curriculum developed by nursing faculty has an organizing framework from which course objectives and learning activities flow in a logical progression over the length of the program" (p. 13). Further guidance is given in the statement "A curriculum design that reflects an organizing framework which provides the basis for program planning, implementation, and evaluation, identifies educational objectives; and drives selection of the content, scope, and sequencing of course work" (p. 15).

Curriculum design in nurse-midwifery is based on the American College of Nurse-Midwives' Core Competencies, which were first developed in 1978 and revised in 1985, 1992, 1997, and 1999; Guidelines and Standards for Practice, developed in 1972 with revisions in 1979, 1987, 1990, and 1993, and the American College of Nurse-Midwives Division of Accreditation (1999) Policies and Procedure Manual for the Practice and Accreditation of Educational Programs in Nurse-Midwifery and Midwifery.

Program Outcomes

A central focus of curriculum design is the stated learning outcomes. The term *outcomes* is the terminology of choice in this book. The authors acknowledge that the term *instructional objectives* can be defined as learner outcomes (Gronlund & Linn, 1995). As already indicated, the term *behavioral objectives* and its use in program criteria by the National League for Nursing was strongly criticized by some proponents of the "curriculum revolution." Concern was expressed that the concept of behavioral objectives supported technical training, was appropriate for some aspects of nursing education, but was inappropriate as the sole approach to professional education. For a number of years a movement parallel to the curriculum revolution was taking place in higher education. This movement was related to assessment of learning. As a result of in-depth study and acceptance of new paradigms, competency based goals and outcomes began to replace the term behavioral objectives. Nurse scholars, in the forefront of this movement, were instrumental in having a draft document promulgated by the National League for Nursing in 1996 using the term outcomes. The 1999 Standards and Criteria (NLNAC) use as a basis for program planning and evaluation "required outcomes" and "elective outcomes." The "program outcomes" determine content, learning experiences, teaching methods, and assessment of learning that has taken place (NLNAC, 1999).

Course Description

The course description is the core document at the course level. It is a detailed description that clearly gives the intent and expectations of the course. The course description serves as a basis for the course outcomes that contribute to the program outcomes. Course outcomes and competencies are the basis for the didactic and clinical assessment of the learner. In addition to giving direction to the content contained in the course outline, they also serve as clear guidelines for the learner as to what s/he must know and do in order to meet the program criteria for graduation and certification. Taken together, all course outcomes define the totality of the learning needed to meet the program outcomes.

Competency Outcomes

Advanced practice nursing and midwifery require an integrated instructional approach. Hence the course competency outcomes include the essential knowledge base and experiences in which the knowledge is applied. The theoretical and clinical competencies are not developed in isolation from each other but rather developed as a unit. Placement of the different practice experiences are determined by the curriculum design.

The development of competency outcome statements is a skill that is readily acquired with practice. A competency outcome statement can be a knowledge, skill, or behavior. Key principles that are inherent in all educational learning outcomes, irrespective of the nomenclature used, follow:

1. It is always learner centered.
2. It is introduced with an action/behavioral verb that describes the expected outcome.
3. It has a time frame.
4. Words used are clear and discreet with a precise meaning.
5. Each outcome must be able to be objectively assessed.
6. Behaviors selected to assess competency are the essential elements that must be known or mastered.
7. Competency outcomes for didactic learning for advanced practice should be written at the higher levels of the taxonomy of the cognitive domain.
8. All domains—cognitive, psychomotor, and affective are included in the competency outcome statements.

What Is Meant by Taxonomy?

Reference has been made to writing competency outcomes at the higher levels of the taxonomy of the cognitive domain. You may be asking, "What is a taxonomy?" Taxonomy is a classification. Bloom and his colleagues classified the cognitive domain in the *Taxonomy of Educational Objectives: Handbook 1. Cognitive Domain*. Their work classifies knowledge in six successive levels of knowing: knowledge, comprehension, application, analysis, synthesis, and evaluation (Bloom et al., 1956). In each successive level the lower level(s) is/are subsumed. Descriptions of each level and suggested use of verbs for use in outcome statements are well developed in *Handbook 1*. The *Taxonomy of Educational Objectives: Handbook 2. Affective Domain* classifies the affective domain in five levels: receiving, responding, valuing, organizing, and characterizing of a value or value complex (Krathwohl, Bloom, & Masia, 1964). Outcomes in the cognitive and affective domain specify the behavior a learner must demonstrate in order that the educator can infer that the outcome has been attained. Since learning cannot be seen, inferences must be made from evidence that can be seen and measured. There is a tendency to give less attention to the affective domain in outcome statements. One reason for this oversight may be the difficulty in the identification of evidence in this domain. If the educator believes the concepts of human caring, empowerment, etc., are core components for advanced nursing education, this must be reflected in the outcomes.

Several taxonomies have been developed for the psychomotor domain. The taxonomy developed by Dave (1970) has been adopted by a number of nurse educators. This taxonomy classifies the progression of attaining a skill in five levels: imitation, manipulation, precision, articulation, and naturalization.

Gronlund (2000) provides a detailed guide for writing instructional objectives. His work includes descriptions of the major categories and illustrative verbs for the cognitive, affective, and psychomotor domains. The chapter on writing higher level thinking skills objectives addresses the cognitive and affective domain. Competency outcomes are also ably presented in the work of Lenburg (1991, 1999).

Course Content and Development

Overall program content is derived from the National Organization of Nurse Practitioner Faculties guidelines and is consistent with required competencies in the specific professional area of nurse practitioner practice and the American College of Nurse-Midwives core competencies. Each individual course uses the conceptual framework, is part of a whole, and contributes to the integrity of the program. Competency outcomes (theory and practice) for each course determine the specific content for the course. The learner attains the competency outcome through a variety of teaching/learning strategies including required readings in hard copy and electronic formats.

Organization of courses is a curriculum decision using the principles of sequence, continuity, and integration. Learning activities, appropriate to the level of the learner, are identified for each course. Teaching methods and strategies and means of assessment are identified and documented for each course. These areas of the curriculum design are presented in chapters 9, 10, and 11. The goal of the curriculum design is to facilitate student achievement of expected outcomes.

SUMMARY

Curriculum development is a learned process. It is a dynamic and very creative process. It is a response to advances in nursing and midwifery knowledge and to the health care needs of society. Although developed to meet the needs as identified at the time of the initial development or revision, it must have sufficient flexibility to incorporate emerging evidence-based educational and clinical practice research. A curriculum should never be a static document. Ongoing course and program evaluation is the basis for curriculum revision.

REFLECTIONS

Bring to mind your nursing and midwifery education program. Are you able to identify specific concepts that provided a framework for the curriculum? How did this framework influence your educational experience? How did it influence your practice?

REFERENCES

American College of Nurse-Midwives. (1997). *Core competencies for basic midwifery practice.* Washington, DC: Author.

American College of Nurse-Midwives Division of Accreditation. (1999). *Policies and procedure manual for the practice and accreditation of educational programs in nurse-midwifery and midwifery.* Washington, DC: Author.

Bevis, E. (1973). *Curriculum building in nursing: A process.* St. Louis: The C. V. Mosby Company.

Bevis, E. (1982). *Curriculum building in nursing: A process* (3rd ed.). St. Louis: The C. V. Mosby Company.

Bevis, E. (1988). New directions for a new age. In *Curriculum revolution: Mandate for change* (pp. 27–52). New York: National League for Nursing.

Bevis, E. (1989). Nursing curriculum as a professional education: Some underlying theoretical models. In E. Bevis & J. Watson (Eds.), *Toward a caring curriculum: A new pedagogy for nursing* (pp. 67–106). New York: National League of Nursing.

Bloom, B. S. (Ed.). (1956). *Taxonomy of educational objectives: Handbook I: Cognitive domain.* New York: David McKay.

Carper, B. A. (1978). Fundamental patterns of knowing in nursing. *Advances in Nursing Science, 1*(1), 13–23.

Chinn, P., & Jacobs, M. (1983). *Theory and nursing: A systematic approach.* St. Louis: C. V. Mosby Company.

Conley, V. C. (1973). *Curriculum and instruction in nursing.* Boston: Little, Brown and Company.

Dave, R. H. (1970). Psychomotor levels. In R. J. Armstrong (Ed.), *Developing and writing behavioral objectives.* Tucson, AZ: Educational Innovators Press.

Diekelmann, N. (1988). Curriculum revolution: A theoretical and philosophical mandate for change. In *Curriculum revolution: Mandate for change* (pp. 137–157). New York: National league for Nursing.

Donaldson, S. K., & Crowley, D. M. (1978). The discipline of nursing. *Nursing Outlook, 26,* 113–120.

Fawcett, J. (1984). *Analysis and evaluation of conceptual models of nursing* (2nd ed.). Philadelphia: F. A. Davis.

Fawcett, J. (2000). *Analysis and evaluation of contemporary nursing knowledge: Nursing models and theories.* Philadelphia: F. A. Davis.

Gronlund, N. (2000). *How to write and use instructional objectives* (6th ed.). Upper Saddle River, NJ: Merrill.

Gronlund, N., & Linn, R. (1995). *Measurement and evaluation in teaching* (6th ed.). New York: Macmillan Publishing Company.

Heidgerken, L. (1953). *Teaching and learning in schools of nursing.* Philadelphia: J. B. Lippincott.

Johnson, D. E. (1980). The behavioral system model for nursing. In J. P. Riehl & C. Roy (Eds.), *Conceptual models for nursing practice* (pp. 207–216). New York: Appleton-Century-Crofts.

King, I. M. (1981). *A theory for nursing systems, concepts, process.* New York: John Wiley & Sons.

Krathwohl, D. R., Bloom, B. S., & Masia, B. B. (1964). *Taxonomy of educational objectives: Book II: Affective domain.* New York: Longman.

Lenburg, C. B. (1991). Assessing the goals of nursing education: Issues and approaches to evaluation outcomes. In M. Garbin (Ed.), *Assessing educational outcomes* (pp. 25–52). New York: National League for Nursing.

Lenburg, C. B. (1999). The framework, concepts and methods of the competency outcomes and performance assessment. *Journal of Issues in Nursing, 4*(2) [On-line]. Available: http://www.nursingworld.org/topic10/tpc10_2.htm

McNeil, J. D. (1985). *Curriculum: A comprehensive introduction.* Boston: Little Brown.

Murdock, J. (1983). Curriculum development in nursing: Historical perspective. In M. B. White (Ed.), *Curriculum development from a nursing model: The crisis theory framework* (pp. 1–25). New York: Springer Publishing.

National League for Nursing Accrediting Commission. (1999). *Accreditation, standards and criteria for academic quality of post secondary and higher degree programs in nursing* [On-line]. Available: htpp://www.accrediting-comm-nlnac.org/

Neuman, B. (1982). *The Neuman's systems model. Application to nursing education and practice.* Norwalk, CT: Appleton-Century-Crofts.

Orem, D. E. (1985). *Nursing: Concepts of practice.* New York: McGraw-Hill.

Riehl, J. P. (1980). Nursing models in current use. In J. P. Riehl & C. Roy (Eds.), *Conceptual models for nursing practice* (2nd ed., pp. 393–398). New York: Appleton-Century-Crofts.

Roy, C. (1984). *Introduction to nursing: An adaptation model.* Englewood Cliffs, NJ: Prentice-Hall.

Taba, H. (1962). *Curriculum development.* New York: Harcourt, Brace and World.

Torres, G., & Lynch, E. (1974). Curriculum process and the integrated curriculum. In *Faculty curriculum development, Part IV, Unifying the curriculum: The integrated approach.* New York: National League for Nursing.

Torres, G., & Stanton, M. (1982). *Curriculum process in nursing: A guide to curriculum development.* Englewood Cliffs, NJ: Prentice-Hall.

Tyler, R. W. (1949). *Basic principles of curriculum and instruction.* Chicago: The University of Chicago Press.

CHAPTER 8

Classroom Teaching Methods and Strategies

We know that the quality of learning is high when students show intellectual, emotional, and ethical growth; we know that teaching is excellent when it fosters such growth, when we have teachers who are willing to care—both about their subjects and for their students.

—L. A. Daloz,
Mentor: Guiding the Journey of Adult Learners

SUGGESTED OUTCOMES FOR THIS CHAPTER

At the completion of this chapter the reader will be able to

1. describe classroom environmental factors conducive to learning;
2. analyze teaching methods for the appropriateness of their use in the education of adults;
3. describe how teaching methods can be selected based on whether the information to be conveyed is in the affective, cognitive, or psychomotor domain.

SETTING THE STAGE FOR LEARNING

Classroom culture affects the learner's ability to learn. Attending to the environment you establish as a teacher requires foresight and planning. There are a number of things to consider in order to ensure an optimum learning environment for students.

Making the expectations and requirements of a course clear to learners is essential at the outset of any course. When possible the learner should participate in setting the goals of the course and these should be discussed at the first class meeting. Having a discussion with learners about their individual goals for the course is a good beginning for this process. Also, it is essential to discuss the applicability of the information or skills to be learned in the course as well as the purpose of each assignment.

There are a number of questions you have to answer for yourself before the course begins. First, you need to consider what assignments you wish to make and the purpose of those assignments. Are there assigned readings? How will the learners demonstrate that they have completed the readings? If one of the assignments is producing a scholarly paper be sure that you are clear with the learner about topic, length, and format. Let learners know what criteria you will use for grading the paper. How much will the grade for the paper influence the course grade? Will there be examinations? What form will they take? How much will they count toward the learner's final grade? Will they be graded on a curve? When will they be given? Once you are clear about all of this, spell it out in the course syllabus that you distribute to the learners, and review it with them on the first day of class.

Concern for the physical comfort of the learners is paramount in establishing a welcoming atmosphere. Be sure to check out the classroom before your first day of class. You don't want any surprises on that first class day. Check the temperature, the lighting, the chairs or desks, chalkboards, and chalk. Be sure to build in break time if your class will be longer than one hour. Tell the learners when they can expect a break and how long it will last. Make sure you start and end on time. Arrive about 5 minutes before class is scheduled to begin so that you are sure you have everything in order. Make the rules of the class clear. Some areas to consider are whether you will allow learners who are late to enter the class, and under what circumstances—should they wait for a break or when acknowledged by the group; whether learners may eat/drink in class; whether they may tape-record the class; whether learners should feel free to get up and walk around the room, or might that be distracting to the group; and whether learners may negotiate a different due date for assignments. Think all of this out ahead of time, and then be sure to make it clear to the learners at the beginning of the course in order to prevent the development of confusion and subsequent problems.

On the first day of class greet the learners with enthusiasm; try to get to know a little bit about each of them. Learn their names as quickly as possible and address them by name. Take some time and have them introduce themselves and tell the class a little about themselves. Let them know that you are interested in them as individuals and that you are there to help them be successful. Tell them a little bit about yourself and why you like teaching this particular course. If this is their first course in the program it is helpful to acquaint them with the facilities in the building in which you are holding class as well as making sure they know where the library, bookstore, and other areas are located on campus. By making the class environment welcoming, respectful of the learner, and as comfortable as possible, you can get the course and the learners off to a positive start. You should encourage learners to participate actively in discussion and feel comfortable in voicing a different opinion from the majority. The climate should be one of respect for each individual.

EVALUATING YOUR TEACHING EFFECTIVENESS

As you begin your teaching career, identify an experienced faculty member who is known to be a good teacher and seek her out as a mentor. Observe her teaching in the classroom. Arrange for her to observe your teaching and give you feedback. Depending on where you teach, there may be formal mechanisms in place for peer review. Peer review, a means to assess a colleague's behavior and provide constructive feedback, is often a requirement for faculty teaching in schools of nursing. Peer review can be formative or summative. Formative peer review involves another faculty member observing your teaching and using specific criteria to evaluate your competence. You will then be given this feedback in a supportive way in an attempt to assist you in improving your teaching techniques and your growth and development as a faculty member. In summative peer review you again are evaluated by a faculty member but the evaluation is used in making decisions about contract renewal or promotion and tenure. Appendixes B and C contain sample criteria to use during the peer review process. The faculty who participate in formative and summative peer review may be selected by the school, or by the teacher being evaluated. It depends on the policies of the institution. In order for peer review to be successful it must be objective, faculty must be skilled at observation, constructive feedback must be given, and this must occur in a climate of trust and open communication. Peer evaluation is typically only one component of faculty evaluation. Mechanisms for student evaluations as well as evaluations by division heads or deans may also be in place. As a new teacher it is extremely helpful to get direct feedback about your classroom performance and you would certainly want to get both written and verbal feedback from your students (Brown & Ward-Griffin, 1994; Ciesla & Lovejoy, 1997).

TEACHING METHODS AND ADULT LEARNERS
Lecture

The lecture is perhaps the most familiar teaching method for many learners. Darkenwald and Merriam (1982) reported that it is the most preferred and most used teaching method in adult education. It is a valuable method when you have a large class but without modification it guarantees passivity on the part of the learner. It is often inappropriately used to "deposit" large amounts of information in students' brains. The teacher is the "expert" and the transmitter of information. When conducted in this manner lecturing is an inappropriate method to use with adult learners. Adult learners need to be actively involved in the learning process. Lectures can be modified to ensure learner participation through the use of questioning, small group discussion interspersed with lecture, and individual activities interspersed with lecture (Cravener, 1997; Greenhalgh, 1997). Learners can be given preparatory readings for the class, and the lecture can be used to clarify difficult material that may not be clear from the readings. It should not be used for material that can easily be understood and learned through reading. This method is appropriate when your objectives for the class are cognitive (Oddi, 1983). Lectures are useful in helping students develop and apply concepts, generalize from knowledge already learned, and practice problem solving skills (Jones, 1984). Research conducted on the lecture method reveals that it is as effective as other methods for presenting information and providing explanations but problem solving skills are taught more effectively in small groups (Beard & Hartley, 1984; Bligh, 2000; Dunkin, 1983).

When planning a lecture first clarify what it is you want the students to know at the end of your time together. Decide what concepts you will have to cover in order to accomplish your objectives. Then you will need to make a detailed outline for yourself, even though you will not be *reading* your lecture. If you have gone over a difficult concept, summarize it before going on to another concept. You may want to read the lecture material aloud to yourself so that you can estimate how much time it will take to deliver the material. Most new teachers prepare more material than they can cover in the allotted time so plan what you will do if you don't get through all the material you prepared. Decide whether you wish to give students an outline to follow along with your lecture or if you want to give them detailed notes. You want to consider the use of audiovisual materials during the class. Some learners are more visual than auditory and having more than one approach helps you reach more learners. Prepare the questions you are going to ask the learners during the lecture. Be sure to have them written down so you may refer to them during the class. Specific questions can be at any cognitive level. You want to ensure that you have questions across all the levels in Bloom's taxonomy. The lower levels of knowledge and comprehension are demonstrated when students recite what they have learned. The higher levels, application, analysis, and synthesis require learners to apply knowledge in specific situations, break down a concept to its components and understand how they work together to produce the whole, and develop new and unique solutions (Wink, 1993).

If you are going to break the class up into small groups for discussion or problem solving based on the material you have presented be sure to estimate the time you will need both for the small group work but also for the small groups to report back to the entire class. Have clear directions for what the group is to accomplish.

Start the class by stating what it is you are going to cover, how the class will be conducted, whether you want to be interrupted by questions or have the learners hold them to the end, about how long you plan to lecture, if there will be group work, problem solving, etc., and when the learners will have a break. Then deliver the material and be sure to summarize at the end.

Observe the class to see if they look like they understand or are confused. Ask them periodically if they comprehend what you are saying. Watch to see if their attention is lagging and be ready to change the pace of your delivery. Learners give many nonverbal cues when they are bored, tired, or uncomfortable. Moving around the room a bit rather than standing rigidly at a podium and varying the pitch of your voice help to keep the learner's attention.

Because adults learn best when they understand how they can use the information presented it is important in APN education to point out the relevance of the class content. Giving examples of clinical application of the information is helpful and also keeps the class's attention. Real life examples are best. The questions you use may be posed as clinical situations and will encourage the learners to develop their clinical thinking skills as well as aid in their understanding of the application of the information. The small work groups could be finding solutions to clinical problems based on the lecture and readings materials. For example, following a lecture on interpreting the CBC (complete blood count), learners could be given actual lab reports as well as subjective data about the client and asked to make a diagnosis.

In summary, lecture is appropriate when your objectives are cognitive, when you want to assist students in understanding complex concepts and their application, and when you want to assist the learner in connecting previous learning with the new concepts.

Group Discussion

Group discussion is indicated when the class objectives are cognitive and/or affective, particularly those concerned with problem solving, concept exploration, and exploration of feelings and beliefs. Careful planning is essential if group discussion is to be successful. Preparing learners by giving them clear objectives for the class and stressing the importance of preparatory work, like readings, videos, or problems to consider, is essential. The physical environment should be conducive to the learners talking with each other. Having the learners sit in a circle so that they can see each other is a helpful technique. The teacher should also sit in the circle and be on the same level as the learners. The size of the group is important. If there are too few members the discussion will lag, with too many members the shyer learners are less likely to speak up. Between 10 and 20 members is what many consider an optimum size for group discussion (Brookfield, 1990).

The role of the teacher in a group discussion is that of facilitator. Rather than imparting information you assist the learners in verbalizing what they know, think, or feel. Setting the ground rules for the discussion and ensuring that learners understand them should occur before the discussion starts. There are a number of ground rules you can consider. Some examples are learners must be respectful of individuals who hold different opinions or beliefs from their own, no one should monopolize the discussion, and individuals should be allowed to talk without being interrupted. The teacher should speak very little during the discussion. You will need to have some questions or statements prepared to get the discussion started or to move it along if it stagnates. An opening question to start the discussion should allow for several different correct answers. A question that deals with opinions would fall into this category. (For example: Do you think oral contraceptives should be sold without a prescription?) Don't be tempted to fill in silent periods by talking. Sometimes learners need some time to think about the discussion before they go on. Also, that silent period may encourage one of the quieter members of the group to participate. Other functions of the teacher in a group discussion are redirecting the group if it strays too far from the topic at hand, keeping anyone from monopolizing the discussion, encouraging more silent members of the group to talk, making sure that the tone of the discussion is respectful and that learners are not ridiculed if they hold a divergent opinion, and summarizing the discussion at the end. At the same time the teacher has to be attuned to the emotional tone of the group. It is important to acknowledge feelings of anger, sadness, frustration, and fear that students may experience. If the emotional tone is not acknowledged it is difficult for learning to take place. Facilitating a group discussion can be very challenging. It is helpful for a beginning teacher to observe someone who is skilled in facilitating group discussions.

In evaluating the group discussion session it is important to determine whether critical thinking on the part of the participants occurred. This does not have much to do with how much discussion took place but rather the quality of the discussion. Long periods of silence may be indicative of thoughtful pauses necessary for critical thought and should not automatically be viewed as a sign of failure.

Group discussion is an excellent method for adult learning. It recognizes the value of the learner's past experiences and current knowledge. It requires that learners be active in the learning process. It increases the learners' group interaction skills. In many ways it is particularly relevant to APN and midwifery education. It allows for discussion of alternative treatment plans and their rationale. It is an excellent vehicle for discussion of the many ethical issues presented in primary care and midwifery. It allows learners to use previous nursing knowledge in new and challenging ways. It allows less experienced learners to benefit from more experienced nurses' knowledge.

Seminar

A seminar is a learner-led group discussion. One learner or a group of learners may be responsible for the class. In addition to allowing active participation of learners it allows the learners to assume the role of facilitator, and to develop skill in group technique and interpersonal skills. It also allows the learner experience in researching materials, writing objectives, and organizing a learning experience. The learner does not accomplish this in isolation but in consultation with the teacher. If the subject is preselected the learner should research the topic and meet with the faculty with the beginning formulation of objectives for the course and a suggested reading list. The faculty member can guide the learner to resources that s/he may have overlooked and can assist in refining the class objectives. Faculty can assist learners in the development and/or use of audiovisual materials. Finally, the learner should have an outline of concepts to be covered in the class and some introductory questions as discussion starters. A reading list should be distributed to the rest of the class at least one week before the scheduled seminar in order to allow sufficient time for the other learners to prepare for the class. The teacher's role when the class takes place is to evaluate the process of the class, what the leaders of the seminar are doing, and the participation and cooperation of the other members of the class. Self-evaluation by the leaders of the seminar should be accomplished at the end of the class as well as evaluation by the other class members.

For APN and midwifery education an interesting case from the learner's clinical experience could be the starting point for the seminar. It is particularly meaningful if it is a case in which more than one action would be appropriate or one that requires ethical decision-making. This approach would help learners develop clinical decision-making skills, improve their ability to argue their clinical approach to a problem, and develop interpersonal skills.

Case Study

The use of the case study meets many of the learner's needs in adult education. It draws on the past experience of the learner, is participatory in nature, and requires the learner to be active. It also builds new knowledge on previous knowledge and experience, allows learners to benefit from each other's knowledge and experience, increases individuals' critical thinking skills, and allows learners to see the way others think. Furthermore, in the education of APNs and midwives it allows for immediate clinical application based on real life situations of new concepts and information, and helps the learner in the development of clinical decision-making skills. We have found the use of case studies to be invaluable in the education of APNs and midwives. An entire class session can be built around a particular case; learners or the teacher can be the facilitator. Cases can be used at the end of a lecture in order to clarify the clinical application of new concepts. Cases can also be used as examinations or as assignments. They can be utilized to meet both cognitive and affective objectives.

Designing cases for use is a time-consuming and sometimes difficult endeavor. Some cases are based on a particular actual patient/client situation; some are a combination of different patient/client situations. We have found it helpful to have other APNs and midwives review the cases we write for clarity and relevance before giving them to students. The content must be clear and well organized. It is helpful to organize it in the same way one would find the information in a medical record. Start with the subjective data, then the objective data. You can include results of diagnostic studies as well as the physical examination. The learner should then list what other information they wish they had in the investigation of the case, and their plan. We have found it helpful to have learners divide their plan into diagnostic studies—ones they believe should have also been ordered, therapeutics, patient education, and follow-up. If you want to increase the learner's knowledge of billing, insurance, and cost of health care, you can require learners to include CPT (Current Procedural Terminology) codes and the cost of any other diagnostic studies and medications. The analysis of and discussion of the case can be facilitated by the faculty or one or more of the learners. We have found it helpful for faculty to lead the analysis and discussion of the first two or three cases of the semester, modeling for learners an approach to the process. We then have the learners, in pairs, lead the discussions of subsequent cases. They are required to cite research-based articles for the rationale for the approach they take to the clinical problems. Learners who have a different approach are also required to cite research-based articles to support their approach. Since cases can be written at varying levels of complexity they can be used with any level of learner.

Gaming

Using games for teaching specific topics fits well with adult learning theory. Games allow learners to share their knowledge and be active participants in the teaching/learning process. Games are an excellent technique to use when wanting to review a large body of knowledge and allow for reinforcement of facts, or when the topic is dry, concrete, and boring to teach in other formats. In addition, gaming can be fun for both learners and faculty. Although they can be fun to implement, games like other teaching techniques require meticulous preparation.

The instructor must consider the type of knowledge to be learned and determine what the desired objectives and outcomes of the game are to be. Knowledge in the cognitive domain lends itself most favorably to the technique of gaming. Examples of topics which lend themselves to this technique in advanced practice nursing education include various physiology topics, family planning information, physical assessment knowledge, and sexually transmitted diseases. The cognitive aspects of these and other topics can be taught or reviewed using gaming.

Games can be individually focused and used as assignments or can be participative and take place during class time. An example of individually focused games are puzzles such as crossword puzzles or word finds. Examples of participative games are board games, such as Trivial Pursuit, Jeopardy, and Bingo. An overview of a number of available previously developed games on nursing topics can be found in an article by Merrily A. Kuhn in the January/February 1995 edition of *The Journal of Continuing Education in Nursing* (Kuhn, 1995). A number of researchers have studied the use of games as a teaching technique and have found them to be very successful (Ball, 2000; Burns, 1984; Henry, 1996; Kramer, 1995; Lewis, Saydak, Mierzwa, & Robinson, 1989; Resko & Chorba, 1992; Sisson & Becker, 1988).

Just as in test construction, careful construction of the questions used in the game is essential as is keeping a record of the source for the answer to individual questions. There should be only one right answer to the question. Determination, explanation, and strict adherence to the rules of the game are essential for success. Trying out the gaming technique on colleagues before implementing it in the classroom can help you avoid mistakes in construction and implementation. Gathering all necessary equipment and assuring it is functional must be accomplished just prior to implementation. It is often helpful to have token prizes for participants and winners. Tape measures, vision testing cards, and pregnancy wheels are examples of prizes that drug companies may be willing to donate to make the game even more fun. As in all teaching methods careful evaluation of this technique is imperative. Faculty and learner evaluation should be accomplished at the close of the game.

Simulation, Role-Playing, Guided Imagery

These three teaching methodologies are appropriate when the content to be taught is in the affective domain. All require the learner to get in touch with feelings about certain patients or patient situations. Role-playing can be used to have the learners assume the role of a particular patient from a socially and medically disenfranchised group that typically experiences some level of discrimination in our health care system. Acting out the role of these patients in a carefully constructed, realistic scenario often provides insight that previously was not present to the learner. Simulation accomplishes much the same as role-playing and requires the learner to deal with a real life situation that they may never have been exposed to. Simulation, unlike role-playing and guided imagery, can be used successfully in acquisition of psychomotor skill through the use of simulated models or computerized simulations of patient situations.

Guided imagery requires the learner to get in touch with often unconscious feelings and reactions to unfamiliar situations. It can be defined as "a purposeful, time limited exercise during which participants are encouraged to relax and focus attention on thoughts, feelings, sensations, sights and sounds evoked by a specific situation described by the guide" (Tuyn, 1994, p. 157). The reflections produced through guided imagery can remain private or be shared with classmates.

DISTANCE LEARNING AND ADVANCED PRACTICE NURSING EDUCATION AND MIDWIFERY

Distance learning is not a new concept. Home study courses were available over the radio and through what were known as correspondence courses long before computers and interactive video was available. Today, off-campus courses range from the paper and pencil correspondence courses to high-tech interactive video conferencing.

Distance education meets many of the philosophical goals of adult education. It allows learners freedom to access courses at a time convenient for them and requires them to be self-directed. Historically, distance education has been used to extend educational opportunities to rural or isolated sites. Now, however, distance education is used to make educational opportunities available to individuals who would have difficulty fitting into their lives the typical educational schedule of classes.

Distance education can take many forms; self-instructional packets, web-based courses, or live two-way video and two-way audio format. Typically, distance education is divided into modalities that are synchronous or asynchronous. Synchronous education refers to communication that is immediate. It is often referred to as "live." Asynchronous education implies a delay between the sending and receiving of information (Lewis, 2000).

Asynchronous Distance Education

The strength of asynchronous distance education is that it does not require the learner to be present at a specific time. It also encourages learner centered learning. The learner controls the order of the material and the time spent on specific topics. Content can be delivered through paper and pencil materials, audiotapes, videotapes, or web-based course content. Web-based content is most commonly used today and it is what we will focus on.

Learners must possess computer skills to participate and need to know what the hardware requirements are for the course. In addition, they should have some familiarity with the Internet and Internet access from wherever they will participate.

Faculty must be enthusiastic about conducting asynchronous distance education if it is to be successful. They must have basic computer literacy skills and an understanding of web-based technology. Technical support is essential in order for faculty to learn to manage software packages that are designed for course construction. Course preparation is time-consuming. In addition to working with the course software and inputting the necessary information, arrangements must be made for mailing required texts to students and arranging access to library materials. Reconceptualization of content and delivery methods is essential in order to adapt traditional classroom environment to a virtual electronic classroom.

There are a number of software programs for course design and most contain a mechanism for E-mail, a mechanism for either a chat room or a bulletin board, a secure area for depositing assignments and exams, and the course content. A bulletin board allows the learners and faculty to post messages to each other to be read when the learner or faculty are on-line. A chat room requires participants be on-line at the same time and communication occurs through posting messages that are read and responded to immediately by others in the chat room. In addition to faculty being available by E-mail and through chat rooms or bulletin boards, it is helpful to be available by phone for students who are experiencing problems and need some direct personal contact.

Learners are able to download the course software from the Internet using a password issued by the school. They then can navigate through the materials at their own pace and utilize the communication avenues available through the program. You may choose to include all of the course materials at the beginning of the course or you can add them as the course goes on. You may choose to have the learners take exams on-line or if you prefer, you can use mailed exams. Learners who previously would not have been able to take courses benefit greatly from the ability to utilize asynchronous distance programs (McHugh & Gibson, 2000).

Synchronous Distance Education

Synchronous distance education can be accomplished in a number of ways. One-way video and two-way audio was perhaps the first model used. This allowed the distant sites to see and hear the instructor but the instructor was unable to see the distant students. Two-way interactive video can allow the instructor and distant sites to see and hear each other but the instructor may only be able to see one distant site at a time. Ideally, the system links an instructor and audience in one classroom to several remote classrooms designated as receiver sites. The instructor and the remote sites can both see and hear each other in real time. The instructor, through any number of large monitors in the transmission site, can simultaneously see the students at all of the distant sites. Interaction can take place at any time. In addition to verbal communication the instructor can make use of video clips, power point presentations, and have the camera focus on written materials. The instructor site can give demonstrations and return demonstrations can be given by the remote sites.

In order to facilitate transmission a technician must be present at each site. S/he is responsible for adjusting equipment as necessary and for troubleshooting. It is important to keep the technician informed of what you are going to do so that s/he has all the necessary equipment and is ready to adjust cameras or do whatever is necessary. Meeting with the technician prior to transmission time and going over your plan for the class will help ensure that all goes smoothly.

Meticulous advance preparation is essential if synchronous distance education is to be successful. Students must receive course materials either through the mail or via E-mail or the World Wide Web prior to the start of the course. Library access, access to texts, and an established method of communication outside of transmission time must be established prior to the course. Reconceptualizing course content to fit the transmission model of delivery is essential. If transmission time is scheduled it is imperative to start and end on time. Video-taping of each session ensures that if transmission difficulties occur those students who were unable to see or hear the transmission have a backup method for receiving the content of the class.

Concern about making distant students feel part of the course is important when utilizing distance education. Some schools have employed adjunct faculty as site coordinators. They are present during each transmission and available to students at other times for problems, concerns, or encouragement. Other schools have had the course faculty visit the distant sites to meet and interact with the students. Learning the distant students' names and addressing them by name during transmissions helps them feel a part of the class. Some schools have highly developed sites and can transmit from the distant classrooms. Having the faculty rotate through the distant sites and transmit from them helps the distant students feel more actively involved in the course.

REFLECTIONS

Think about the learning experiences you have had that have made you feel most participative and involved in the teaching/learning process. What teaching methods did the instructor use that drew you into the topic and involved you in the class?

Have you tried using those methods in your own teaching? Is there material you are currently teaching that would lend itself to those methods?

REFERENCES

Ball, K. (2000). Anatomy and physiology: Games we play. *Nurse Educator, 25*(4), 156–157.

Beard, R., & Hartley, J. (1984). *Teaching and learning in higher education* (4th ed.). London: Harper and Row.

Bligh, D. (2000). *What's the use of lectures?* 1st U. S. ed. San Francisco: Jossey-Bass.

Brookfield, S. D. (1990). Discussion. In M. W. Galbraith (Ed.), *Adult learning methods: A guide for effective instruction* (pp. 187–204). Malabar, FL: Krieger.

Brown, B., & Ward-Griffin, C. (1994). The use of peer evaluation in promoting nursing faculty teaching effectiveness: A review of the literature. *Nurse Education Today, 14,* 299–305.

Burns, K. (1984). Experience in the use of gaming and simulation as an evaluation tool for nurses. *The Journal of Continuing Education in Nursing, 15,* 213–217.

Ciesla, J. S., & Lovejoy, N. C. (1997). Peer review a method for developing faculty leaders. *Nurse Educator, 22,* 41–47.

Cravener, P. A. (1997). Promoting active learning in large lecture classes. *Nurse Educator, 22*(3), 21–25.

Daloz, L. A. (1999). *Mentor: Guiding the journey of adult learners,* 2nd ed. San Francisco: Jossey-Bass.

Darkenwald, G. G., & Merriam, S. B. (1982). *Adult education: Foundations of practice.* New York: Harper and Row.

Dunkin, M. J. (1983). A review of research on lecturing. *Higher Education Research and Development, 2,* 63–78.

Edmondson, K. M. (1994). Concept maps and the development of cases for problem-based learning. *Academic Medicine, 69*(2), 108–110.

Greenhalgh, T. (1997). Let's learn more in lectures. *British Medical Journal, 314*(7088), 1207–1208.

Heliker, D. (1994). Meeting the challenge of the curriculum revolution: Problem-based learning in nursing education. *Journal of Nursing Education, 33,* 45–47.

Henry, M. B. (1996). Encore performance: Discovering new directions in gaming. *Journal of Nursing Staff Development, 12*(6), 306–310.

Jones, L. C. (1984). *Teaching primary care nursing.* New York: Springer Publishing.

Kramer, N. (1995). Using games for learning. *The Journal of Continuing Education in Nursing, 33*(3), 137–138.

Kuhn, M. A. (1995). Gaming: A technique that adds spice to learning? *The Journal of Continuing Education in Nursing, 26*(1), 35–39.

Lewis, D., Saydak, S., Mierzwa, L., & Robinson, J. (1989). Gaming a teaching strategy for adult learners. *The Journal of Continuing Education in Nursing, 20*(2), 80–84.

Lewis, J. M. (2000). Distance education foundations. In J. Novotny (Ed.), *Distance education in nursing* (pp. 4–22). New York: Springer Publishing.

McHugh, M. L., & Gisbon, R. (2000). Teaching a web-based course: Lessons from the front. In J. Novotny (Ed.), *Distance education in nursing* (pp. 23–42). New York: Springer Publishing.

Oddi, L. (1983). The lecture: An update on research. *Adult Education Quarterly, 33*(4), 222–229.

Resko, D., & Chorba, M. (1992). Enhancing learning through the use of games. *Dimensions of Critical Care Nursing, 11*(1), 173–176.

Sisson, P., & Becker, L. (1988). Using games in nursing education. *Journal of Nursing Staff Development, 4*(4), 146–151.

Wink, J. (2000). *Critical pedagogy: Notes from the real world* 2nd ed. New York: Longman.

CHAPTER 9

Assessing Learner Progress in the Classroom

Assessment of student learning requires the use of a number of techniques for measuring achievement. But assessment is more than a collection of techniques. It is a systematic process that plays a significant role in effective teaching. It begins with the identification of learning goals and ends with a judgment concerning how well those goals have been reached.

—R. L. Linn and N. E. Gronlund,
Measurement and Assessment in Teaching (8th ed.)

SUGGESTED OUTCOMES FOR THIS CHAPTER

At the completion of this chapter the reader should be able to

1. recognize the importance of developing test questions based on stated outcomes,
2. apply principles of test item construction to multiple-choice questions, and
3. carry out an item analysis for a multiple-choice test for a small group of learners.

INTRODUCTION

The goal of advanced practice programs is to prepare a knowledgeable and competent practitioner who is capable of providing safe and effective care for a specific population. It is the responsibility of both the learner and the educator to validate that the knowledge, skills, and attitudes documented in the curriculum statements of competency outcomes have been attained. This requires the development of assessment tools that 1) are objective and capable of assisting the learner and educator to make a judgment and 2) can attest that the desired level of competency has been demonstrated. This chapter will briefly review assessment and describe classroom testing as one means of assessing the knowledge base of the practitioner.

THE ASSESSMENT PROCESS

Assessment is a general term that includes the full range of procedures used to gain information about student learning and the formation of value judgments concerning learner progress (Linn & Gronlund, 2000). Educational assessment, as a process, is a means used to determine the effectiveness of teaching and/or determining the value of a learning experience in assisting the learner to achieve the expected outcomes of the instruction, course, or program (Conley, 1973; Oermann & Gaberson, 1998). The goal of the assessment process is to enable the learner and educator to gain information related to the degree to which the outcome has been achieved. Westmeyer (1988) presents assessment under two major aspects of learner progress—achievement and performance. Achievement, using Westmeyer's terminology, is related to demonstration of acquired knowledge or information and performance is related to demonstration of expected skills.

Assessment is meant to be a positive experience. The assessment process has the components of formative assessment and summative assessment. Formative assessment is the designated period of time during which guidance and feedback is given to the learner and is not associated with a grade. Formative assessment and self-assessment assist the learner to identify strategies to attain the expected outcomes. A clear understanding of the formative assessment process contributes to a positive learning experience. Summative assessment takes place at a specific point in time when a measurement takes place in relation to the expected outcome and is associated with a grade. There can be several summative points in the course.

There are a variety of tests and strategies for classroom learning measurement. These provide information and are usually objective. It is important to recognize that in assessment one is making a value judgment about the measurement.

Basic to achievement and performance assessment are clearly stated outcomes. These will minimize subjectivity. Misunderstandings are more apt to occur when the learner does not have a clear understanding of the expected outcomes, the criteria to be used, or the methodology used for the summative assessment. Course outlines should include the expected outcomes as well as criteria for class activities, assignments, and methods of assessment. The program materials, distributed to each student, should include defined policies in relation to the grading system and grade requirement for progression in the program.

ACHIEVEMENT TEST DEVELOPMENT

A test is a valuable educational tool that serves several purposes. The primary purpose is to enable the educator to assess if the learner is achieving the stated outcomes. It can also be an indicator of teacher effectiveness in presenting the material. For the learner, results of the test can be motivation for learning as they can give indicators of what has been learned and what areas need additional concentration.

The achievement test should adequately sample the content identified in the course plan to meet the outcomes of the instruction. Many of the outcomes can be measured by a paper and pencil test. The first task in test development is to identify what competency outcomes can be measured by a paper and pencil test and which must be assessed by other techniques. To ensure that the test will adequately measure the selected learning outcomes and course content a table of specifications is developed (Gronlund, 2000). The table of specifications, also known as a test blueprint or grid, is a two dimensional chart. The cells of the vertical dimension represent the outcomes and content to be covered by the test and the intersecting cells of the horizontal dimension, using the taxonomy of the cognitive domain, indicate the level in the cognitive domain that the item is testing. A decision is made on what proportion of the test will be allocated to each outcome and content area. The decision can be made by stating the total number of items for each content area, or percentage of test items allocated to each content area. Ideally, the table of specifications to be of greatest benefit should be prepared before beginning the instructional process and before constructing the paper/pencil test.

Gronlund proposes that for classroom testing, using the number of items may be sufficient, but the percentages are useful in determining the amount of emphasis to give to each area (2000, p. 145). Because of the nature of the professions of nursing and midwifery it is valuable to have one column added to the table to document which outcome(s) have aspects of the affective domain. It may not be possible to have a specific item for each, but it is a constant reminder of the importance of incorporating the affective domain in the expected outcomes and teaching.

A Table of Specifications is shown in Appendix D for a unit on Management of the Care of the Essentially Normal Newborn. The competency outcomes for the unit are: At the completion of the unit the learner will be able to competently 1) integrate a scientific knowledge base to develop and carry out a neonate management plan for the immediate physiologic adjustment to extrauterine life;

2) identify normal characteristics and deviations from the normal during the immediate and ongoing evaluation of the newborn; 3) develop a theoretical framework for maintenance of infant nutritional status; 4) identify specific content and rationale for timing of instructions to parents for infant care; 5) explain anatomic/physiologic basis, differential diagnosis, and nurse-midwifery management including parent counseling, for common problems of the neonate; 6) analyze the problem of neonatal jaundice; and 7) explain deviations from the normal immune response in neonates and implications for neonate health. The table includes 5 levels of the cognitive domain and a column for the affective domain.

One of the responsibilities of the educator is to ensure that the advanced nurse and midwifery practitioner has been provided with opportunities to develop knowledge and skills to promote critical thinking and clinical decision-making. Test items at the lower levels of the cognitive domain do not assess these abilities. The importance of developing instructional outcomes that address analysis, synthesis, and evaluation cannot be overemphasized. Test items must reflect the program expectation of the advanced practitioner.

Test Types

Tests are commonly classified as objective and subjective tests. An objective test is one in which equally competent scorers will obtain the same scores, whereas a subjective test is one in which the scores are influenced by the opinion or judgment of the person doing the scoring (Linn & Gronlund, 2000).

All tests have advantages and disadvantages. The essay test, characterized as a subjective test, allows the learner to self-select content for the response and organize the response in an essay format. It has the advantage of allowing the learner to respond to a topic in greater depth but also has the disadvantage of sampling a limited amount of course content. Techniques to reduce subjectivity include preparation of a detailed answer plan which is used as a guide when scoring each question, reading all papers before scoring the individual paper, and scoring the same question on each paper before moving to the subsequent question.

The objective test includes multiple choice questions, matching, true and false, and short answer questions. It is very structured and requires of the learner a short restricted answer or the selection of a correct response. The objective test has the advantage of covering more content, ease in scoring and analyzing the answer, and if appropriately developed, can assess learning at the lower and higher levels of the cognitive domain. The disadvantage is that unless it is skillfully constructed, it may predominantly measure knowledge at the lower levels of the cognitive domain.

Principles for Writing Questions and Test Items

Although guidelines for the various types of test questions differ, here are some general principles that apply to the construction of all questions and test items.

1. Instructions should be simple and brief.
2. Language should be clear and not ambiguous.
3. All words and content in the question or stem should be essential to the expected response.
4. An answer to a question in the test should not be in the body of another question.

Multiple-Choice Test Items

Key words used for the construction of multiple-choice test items are stem, correct answer or response, and distracters. The stem should have a complete idea and can be a question or a partial sentence. The distracters are the wrong answers or choices. Writing plausible distracters is one of the most difficult aspects in constructing multiple-choice questions. Single test items are independent of each other. Alternately, an item set is context dependent and lends itself to testing a variety of types of complex thinking (Haladyna, 1994). An example of the item set is a vignette with a series of test items based on the content of the vignette. One of the dangers in the item set is inter-item cuing.

Several texts and articles include guidelines for the construction of multiple-choice questions (Haladyna, 1994; Linn & Gronlund, 2000; Oermann & Gaberson, 1998). Some of the key guidelines in these texts follow.

1. State clearly in the instructions whether the choice is the correct answer or best answer.
2. Use plausible or logical distracters.
3. Avoid negative statements but if a negative is used in the stem underline or capitalize it.
4. Be cautious of the use of "none of the above" as a distracter or a correct response.
5. Avoid the use of clues that may suggest the correct answer.
6. Avoid grammatical clues. All options should be grammatically consistent with the stem.
7. Avoid qualifying terms such as "never," "often," "always."

When constructing the test item it is extremely useful to place each item on an individual card, which includes the item and a reference source for the response.

These cards will also be used to document the statistical analysis and over time can serve as a test item bank.

The primary requisite for the construction of appropriate test items is expert knowledge of the educator/clinician in the area to be tested. The actual writing skill is developed with practice and review of the constructed test items with colleagues. For test item construction Haladyna (1994) is a particularly useful reference as he includes a foundation for multiple-choice testing, development of multiple-choice items, and validating test items.

Other Test Formats

Each test format has its own set of rubrics, which are explained in the referenced texts. The completion, short answer, matching, and true-false format are useful for testing factual knowledge (Gronlund, 2000; Haladyna, 1994).

Validity and Reliability

Irrespective of the format of the test, it will not attain its purpose unless the results of the test are valid and reliable. For the test results to be valid the test must measure what it is expected to measure. Development of a table of specifications based on the outcomes and content of the course provides a basis for content and sample validity.

Reliability refers to the consistency of evaluation results. Reliability is concerned with both learner and educator. The classical example for reliability is to give the same classroom test to the same learners on two occasions. If similar scores are obtained it is concluded the test is reliable. This is not practical for classroom testing. A practical approach is teacher ratings as described by Linn and Gronlund: "If different teachers independently rate the same pupils on the same instrument and obtain the same ratings, we can conclude that the results have a high degree of reliability from one rater to another" (2000, p. 74). Oermann and Gaberson describe reliability as the extent to which test scores are accurate, error free, and stable (1998, p. 34).

Test Analysis

A statistical test analysis is a useful tool and can contribute to improved skill in writing multiple-choice questions. Most educational institutions utilize a commercial computerized test analysis program that interprets the score obtained on a large number of variables. The printout gives information on the individual item from all the test papers as well as group statistics. These details are readily available at your educational institution as well as on the World Wide Web. This section will focus on item analysis, with the intent to identify items that can be improved for better testing. It will also describe the non-computer method for analyzing classroom tests for those who do not have access to computerized scoring. There are three pieces of information you want to obtain:

- The item difficulty—was the item an easy or hard item?
- A discrimination index—did the item discriminate between the learners who did well on the test and the learners who did not do well?
- A distracter analysis—which distracters did not work and which worked best?

Selection of the sample of test papers to be included in the analysis is dependent on the class size. Linn and Gronlund (2000) recommend that it is useful for a group of 20 to 40 learners to compare the responses of the 10 highest scorers with the 10 lowest scorers. Groups of 20 and lower should be divided into two groups—the upper half and lower half, while groups over 40 can use the upper and lower 25%. It is important to keep in mind that caution should be taken when interpreting results from a small sized class.

The first step is to record for each item the number of learners that chose each alternate response in the high scoring group and low scoring group. This statistic is the basic figure used in each formula for further calculations.

The item difficulty gives the percent of learners who gave the correct response. *Item Difficulty* formula is $P = 100$ R/T, where P = percentage of students, R = the number of correct responses in the upper and lower groups, and T = the total number of learners in the group who tried the item. Using 28 as the number of correct responses and 40 as the total number of learners the response is 70. R multiplied by 100 divided by T will give the percentage for the item difficulty or 70%. The term "difficulty" can be confusing as the percentage is the number who had the correct response. The point to be remembered is the lower the number is for the item difficulty the more difficult the item was.

The discrimination index discriminates between those who did well on the test and those who did not do well. *Discrimination Index* formula is $D = (RU - RL)/0.5T$. Using the same population with 20 from the upper group getting the correct response and subtracting the number 8 for the number correct in the lower group the figure obtained is 12. This divided by 20, or 1/2 the total group gives a discrimination index of .60. If the high scorers answer the item correctly and low scorers answer incorrectly the discrimination index will be high. An index of > .20 is acceptable.

Distracter Effectiveness can be obtained by a visual examination of the record made for each test item. Distracters that have not been chosen by any person should be revised or eliminated. Distracters are usually difficult to construct. If any one distracter is chosen more often than the correct response, this warrants a more careful analysis of the content of the distracter.

Using statistical measures provides indicators for removal of specific items as well as the improvement of specific items by revising the stem or alternate responses. Skill in item writing is enhanced through the review and revision of test items.

SUMMARY

A variety of paper and pencil tests are available for assessing classroom learning. This chapter has focused on multiple-choice questions. The reader is encouraged to do readings on other formats. Development of test items takes time and should not be left until a few days before the date when the test will be administered. As indicated earlier in this chapter, test items must be based on the stated outcomes and ideally test items should be prepared at the same time that you are preparing the course and lesson plans. If you develop a table of specifications, design the test to cover proportionately those areas of classroom instructions and reading that are deemed most important and have sufficient test items on the total test—the test will have a greater validity. A test should be a motivator and not a dread.

SUGGESTED EXERCISE

If you are in an educational institution take a completed multiple-choice examination and place it in a table of specifications based on the stated outcomes of the unit or course. What changes, if any, would you recommend?

REFERENCES

Conley, V. C. (1973). *Curriculum and instruction in nursing.* Boston: Little, Brown and Company.

Gronlund, N. E. (2000). *How to write instructional objectives* (6th ed.). Englewood Cliffs, NJ: Prentice-Hall.

Haladyna, T. M. (1994). *Developing and validating multiple-choice test items.* Hillsdale, NJ: Lawrence Erlbaum Associates, Publishers.

Linn, R. L., & Gronlund, N. E. (2000). *Measurement and assessment in teaching* (8th ed.). Englewood Cliffs, NJ: Prentice Hall.

Oermann, M. H., & Gaberson, K. B. (1998). *Evaluation and testing in nursing.* New York: Springer Publishing.

Westmeyer, P. (1988). *Effective teaching in adult and higher education.* Springfield, IL: Charles C Thomas.

CHAPTER 10

Teaching in the Clinical Setting

The teacher's "self" is the real instrument of education, and the goal is to develop the student's "self." Once developed as a characteristic, passion will transcend cause, from education to practice, and will create the boldness required for [health] professionals moving in to the future.

—K. R. Stevens,
"Teaching Vision and Passion"

SUGGESTED OUTCOMES FOR THIS CHAPTER

Teaching in the clinical setting is a challenging opportunity. It is a tremendous responsibility to influence the minds and practice of others as we encourage the learners to grow, to reflect on their own progress of learning, and to think for themselves while maintaining the vision of excellent, high quality, health and illness care (Stevens, 1995; Thompson, 1983). At the end of this chapter, the reader will be able to

1. understand and apply the principles of adult teaching and learning in the clinical setting,
2. identify factors that can influence and detract from learning in the clinical setting, and

3. match appropriate teaching strategies to specific learning needs in the clinical setting.

INTRODUCTION

Stevens (1995) noted that one of the current challenges for teachers in preparing the next generation of health professionals is that many of the positions our graduates will hold in their professional lives do not yet exist. This is why she and the authors agree that one of the main tasks of teaching and learning in an advanced practice discipline is an emphasis on learning how to learn, with repeated opportunities to practice what one is learning (Knowles, 1970). We, the teachers, must be willing to accept that today's knowledge may be tomorrow's historical references, and that if the learner is not supported in learning how to learn, today's knowledge will quickly become obsolete and result in obsolete (and potentially dangerous) practice.

Teaching in the clinical setting, based on teaching and learning theories and strategies, includes one vital component in the environment of learning that is not present in the classroom, pre- or post-conferences, or the Internet. That vital component is the physical presence of the person who is the recipient of health and illness care—the patient(s). (Though the writer has difficulty calling human beings "patients" because of the implied passivity in the term, and she totally refutes the notion that our clients are "consumers" in a market-driven economic sense, the term patient will be used throughout this chapter for ease in understanding who the patient is and how their role as the recipient of health and illness services affects the teaching and learning of advanced practice nurses and midwives.) The presence of another human being in the teacher-learner equation can significantly alter that relationship. Though the safety net of expert clinician (teacher or preceptor) is present, the learner understands fully the need to apply theory learned to the care of real people—whether they be child or adult, male or female, or an entire family. The stakes are high and the rewards of a job well done immense!

As this chapter progresses, it will become apparent that much of the content on teaching and learning in the clinical setting is a reinforcement of what has been written about in earlier chapters. The influence of patients and patient needs must be addressed in the care relationship. In addition, the reader is reminded that preparing advanced practice nurses and midwives goes beyond the generalist preparation of the novice nurse. Autonomous roles inherent in advanced practice require a higher level of accountability for the learner, allow limited margin for errors in judgment, and require the learning to proceed at a fairly rapid rate from novice to advanced practice levels within the context of the educational program (Benner, 1984). In other words, teaching in the clinical setting leads to high quality, cost-efficient health and illness care through the preparation of competent, compassionate, and caring practitioners.

TEACHER PREPARATION

The purpose of clinical teaching is to facilitate the application/transfer of knowledge and understanding to the direct care of patients (Bowling, 1993; Thompson, 1983). The physical move from the classroom and asynchronous teaching methods that facilitate the acquisition of theory to the clinical setting where this theory must be applied is a major step for novice teachers. You may be asking yourself, "How do I prepare for such an important role?" The authors suggest that you begin with an appraisal of yourself—your understanding of the role and expectations of a clinical teacher, your level of clinical proficiency, and your willingness to share the care of patients with a new learner who may be slow or a bit clumsy at first.

Questions often arise about teacher readiness (Can I really do this?) and can be answered by formal preparation for this clinical teaching role before taking it on (Hermann, 1997). Advanced practice nursing or midwifery faculty have a responsibility to offer formal preparation to clinical teachers and this is often done in the form of workshops. Clinical proficiency is a must for the clinical teacher—adult learners will quickly assess your clinical expertise as they are determining whether or not to trust your judgment, and, hence, your role as facilitator and supporter of good clinical care. Understanding the expectations of a clinical teacher, especially if the clinical teacher is not the same as the classroom or theory teacher, is an important step in preparing oneself for teaching in the clinical area. These expectations need to be defined and shared by the academic program faculty and often are written down for easy reference (See chapter 13). Table 10.1 provides a summary of clinical teacher preparation.

TABLE 10.1 Preparation for Clinical Teaching

Review adult learning theories
Understand how adults learn
Review principles of teaching and learning
Know your own strengths and limitations as teacher
Think critically and facilitate critical thinking in others
Maintain theoretical and clinical competence
Know the level of the learner and expectations for performance
Know clinical area—policies, protocols
Plan for clinical experiences
Identify any obstacles for learning in the clinical setting

Clinical teaching goes beyond the direct care of individuals today and pushes both teacher and learner to use principle-based critical thinking that affords flexibility and adaptability to patient needs now and in the future (Evans, 2000; Gaberson & Oermann, 1999). As noted earlier, today's realities of clinical practice may not be tomorrow's, requiring that the clinical teacher encourage and sometimes push the learner to go beyond the preceptor's preferred way of practicing. This reinforces the notion that the clinician-teacher cannot require the learner to do it "the teacher's way" unless there is a solid rationale for doing so and, thus, deliberately overriding the learner's approach to care. Referring back to the chapter on critical thinking, novice learners sometimes expect a recipe for providing care to individuals. This is a very unrealistic expectation and the clinician-teacher must avoid the temptation to give in to this request in the interest of time (it is easier to tell someone what to do rather than wait for them to think it through themselves). "Just tell me how to do it" requests from the novice practitioner must be replaced by encouragement to take a few minutes to reflect on what the learner thinks is going on and help her/him to think through what the best approach might be. It is the role of the clinical teacher to support and promote a learning environment of inquiry and discovery within the learner before they graduate and are on their own for future learning.

TEACHING AND LEARNING IN A CLINICAL SETTING

Over half a century ago, Highet (1950) noted that teaching was inseparable from learning. Today's environment of constant change and challenge suggests that teachers need to fully understand principles of teaching and learning in order to be most effective in their role as clinical teacher—that is, how teaching and learning fit together. In an earlier writing, the author defined *teaching* as "the conscious manipulation of the [learner's] environment in such a way that his or her activities will contribute to his or her development as a person" and clinician (Thompson, 1983, p. 21). *Learning* was defined as "a change in behavior, perception, insights, attitudes, or any combination of these that can be repeated when the need is aroused." Both teaching and learning are dynamic, interactive processes that can positively or negatively influence one another. Good teaching supports learning, and even though formal teaching is not required for learning to take place, learning is clearly the expected goal of teaching.

There are many principles of teaching and learning discussed in the literature related to teaching in a clinical discipline. Several will be discussed here. The reader is encouraged to select those that are most appropriate to the level of learner, domain of learning (cognitive, affective, psychomotor), and environment for learning. Building upon Bevis's (1978) exploration of the progression of learning, the clinical teacher has the primary responsibility to assist and support the learner in transferring acquired knowledge and experience to the clinical setting and care of patients. It is during this operation stage that the learners need time to practice, repeat, and test out their own ideas as they make their knowledge work for them.

As noted by Thompson (1983) and O'Shea (1994), there is much overlap in the principles of learning applicable in both the classroom and clinical settings. However, several principles are especially pertinent to clinical teaching. A selection of such principles of learning will be discussed here briefly, along with suggested teacher behaviors that can guide the choice of teaching methods in the clinical setting.

1. *Learning requires the active participation of the learner:* The teacher must engage the learner as an active participant, avoiding the "telling" mode and encouraging discovery learning.

2. *Learning is more effective when it occurs in response to perceived needs of the learner:* The teacher must understand and support learner needs while also helping the learner to see the connection between knowledge, patient needs, and clinical practice and gently moving the learner to increased levels of self-direction and accountability.

3. *Learning requires understanding:* The teacher must present ideas and concepts clearly, offering alternative explanations as needed, and checking for understanding frequently.

4. *Learning takes time:* Teaching requires patience and the teacher needs to have highly developed skills of listening, watching, and waiting.

5. *Learning is enhanced when one moves from the familiar to the unfamiliar:* The teacher selects clinical experiences that build upon prior learning, moving from simple to complex patient situations.

6. *Learning proceeds at different rates, in different ways, and with different patterns, including periodic plateaus:* The teacher needs to select teaching methods that fit learner needs, patterns of learning, and performance outcomes as learner proceeds from novice to advanced beginner.

7. *Learning is retained longer when it can be put to immediate use:* The teacher offers early and frequent clinical exposure as knowledge is acquired.

8. *Learning is enhanced by repetition:* The teacher provides multiple opportunities to provide patient care and perform psychomotor skills, with appropriate feedback on performance.

9. *Learning must be reinforced:* The teacher encourages self-evaluation of learning with reinforcement of positive learning and correction of errors.

10. *Learning requires known performance outcomes:* The teacher sets boundaries of safe practice, defines expected outcomes of learning, and supports learner achievement of these outcomes.

11.   *Learning is affected by emotions, including the positive effects of mild to moderate anxiety:* The teacher understands the nature of human responses to learning in the clinical setting and creates an environment of trust and mutual respect, relative calm, helpfulness, freedom of expression, and acceptance of different approaches to patient care.

12.   *Learning is easier when the learner sees progress and is successful:* The teacher assists the learner to evaluate progress and offers feedback on progress.

13.   *Learning is facilitated by ideas more than facts:* The teacher encourages critical thinking, principled action, and alternative approaches for patient care supported by sound reasons.

14.   *Self-directed learning and accountability are learned behaviors:* The teacher knows when to step back, and offers multiple opportunities for learner to be accountable for patient care and self-directed in his or her approach to patient care.

15.   *Learning must be satisfying to the learner to maintain motivation for ongoing learning:* The teacher's major responsibility is to teach others how to learn, modeling and reinforcing the need for continued learning throughout one's professional career and life.

There are many articles and books that the clinical teacher can refer to in order to gather data that supports the importance of these principles when teaching in the clinical setting. The reader is referred to the selected bibliography at the end of this chapter for further reading.

FACTORS THAT INFLUENCE CLINICAL LEARNING

Factors that promote learning in the clinical setting range from learner and teacher characteristics to environment and patient needs and/or expectations. If one were to reflect on the best learner they have had or observed, words like able, motivated, prepared, and flexible often come to mind. In addition, a learner who is eager and willing to assume the role and responsibilities inherent in advanced practice nursing or midwifery is a joy to teach, for the learning needs are clearly defined and the learner is fully responsible for their own learning (you do not have to direct and pull the learner along—you need to support and coach [Blanchard, 1985] as the learner moves himself or herself along the path of learning the new practice role). Learners who are willing and able to accurately evaluate their progress in learning while also remaining open to constructive feedback from teachers and peers make the task of clinical teaching easier. In decades of clinical teaching, the author has found the most difficult learner is the one who thinks she knows it all (you cannot teach her anything) or worse, one who lacks insight into his own performance and overrates his progress (very unsafe).

Teacher characteristics that promote learning in the clinical area have been referred to throughout this and other chapters. For example, the teacher must possess up-to-date, expert clinical knowledge and skills, as modeling is crucial to learning the advanced practice role. A teacher who is approachable, patient, respectful, and flexible is rated highly effective by learners in health professional education (Davis, Sawin, & Dunn, 1993; Hayes, 1994; Irby, Ramsey, Gillmore, & Schaad, 1991; O'Shea & Parsons, 1979; Reilly & Oermann, 1992). Motivation, humor, and enjoyment of the teaching role are other positive teacher characteristics that promote learning. The teacher also needs excellent interpersonal skills, including the ability to give both good and bad news in a supportive way. The ability to correctly identify learner differences and needs, and work collaboratively with the learner to achieve expected performance outcomes are other qualities of a good clinical teacher. Knowing when to step in, step back, and step out of the clinical situation are key teacher behaviors that foster clinical growth and competence in new learners (Blanchard, 1985; Rideout, 1994). Likewise, a clinical teacher needs to be able to diagnose learner difficulties or roadblocks to learning, work with the learner to overcome these difficulties, and give appropriate and timely feedback on learner performance. Honesty with caring is vital when learning stops and the learner needs to be counseled to seek another career path—fortunately a relatively rare occurrence in advanced practice nursing and midwifery.

Teacher behaviors that detract from learning in the clinical area include an insistence on "my way" to the exclusion of any alternative thought or approaches in the learner, and the opposite characteristics of those described above as positive. The teacher in the clinical setting can become the greatest barrier to critical thinking in the learner out of a need to control the situation, or out of fear that the learner will make a mistake that will threaten the teacher's relationship with the patient (especially when the teacher-clinician owns the practice where learning is taking place). If the teacher refuses to allow the learner time to learn and experiment with their own thinking about patient care, the learner may stop thinking all together. Taking over clinical decision-making when there is no immediate danger to the client is tantamount to saying to the learner—"You obviously don't know what you are doing!" This teacher approach can undermine the learner's confidence and competence in thinking and practice, suggesting that s/he is not capable of making decisions or providing good care to clients. One of the most common clinical teacher behaviors that limits critical thinking is refusing to listen to a full report on a client before demanding the diagnosis—an impatient "get to the point" directive that suggests that one can make good decisions on incomplete data. The novice clinician begins to think that one can jump to a conclusion without going through a rational process of gathering information, sorting through that information to set priorities, and then deciding what the client's condition or needs are.

Environmental factors that promote learning in a clinical setting include both emotional and physical components. An environment of calmness with minimal distractions allow learning to proceed, even during patient emergencies. It is the teacher's responsibility to remain calm in difficult situations so that learner anxiety is minimized (Massarweh, 1999). Sometimes the teacher has to control distractions, such as blocking the door to a laboring woman's room so that the novice midwifery student can establish rapport with the woman, and proceed with labor management without interference from others (doctors, nurses, other students). The clinical teacher can keep the other professional staff informed of progress of labor and reassure them that if anything changes, she will let them know in a timely manner. Pleasant surroundings and adequate space to care for patients including space with the patient for both learner and clinical teacher contribute to clinical learning. Likewise, an environment that is used to and supportive of health professional education contributes to a positive learning experience. Introduction of health professional learners into a practice that has never had such students before takes lots of planning, explanation, orientation, and patience as the staff adjusts to the learners and their need to do many of the things staff have been used to doing.

The complexity of patient needs can both facilitate and detract from learning. As learning progresses, patients with complex needs can contribute to further learning and clinical competence. However, if the setting requires complex decision-making at all times, it may slow down the learning in a novice (learning proceeds from simple to complex). This latter clinical situation may require that the educational program use more simulated laboratory experiences prior to assigning the learner to the care of actual patients.

Time is always a factor in learning—whether the time needed to perform a skill, think through a patient situation, gather information from the patient, or process that information in order to construct a plan of care or treatment. Time limits on performance need to be clearly stated and progressively shorter as the learner proceeds throughout the educational program. Time during emergency situations is always limited, and here the clinical teacher will often take a more directive-oriented approach to teaching, or take over the actual care until the emergency is under control. Talking about what took place immediately after the emergency helps the learner understand more fully what happened, why it happened, and what role the learner might take the next time such an emergency arises.

Conflicts between the clinical teacher and learner can detract from learning in the clinical setting. These conflicts may be as simple as a genuine difference in style and personality to a more serious conflict in teacher and learner expectations for performance. Hayes (1994) summarizes several sources of conflict in the learner-preceptor relationship. These include differing perceptions of learner readiness to take on role functions and preceptor reluctance to trust the learner to take on increasing responsibility. Other sources of potential conflict include age differences between teacher and learner and the preceptor belief that a learner without previous nursing experience is a "drain" on teaching—it takes too much time to teach them advanced practice skills and therefore they should not be allowed to enter such APN programs. Personality differences are inevitable, but can be overcome as both teacher and learner get to know and understand each other. This takes time, as trust is not automatic in any human relationship. Cultural insensitivity, ignorance, and prejudice should never be tolerated in the teaching-learning or practice environment as such behaviors lead to an intolerable situation for all parties (Snyder & Bunkers, 1994). It falls to the teacher to set the example of appropriate interaction with all people, starting with the learner, and modeling such behaviors in their care of patients as well. A good rule of thumb in all situations is to treat the learner the way you would want to be treated, or at the very best, the way you would treat the patient.

TEACHING STRATEGIES IN THE CLINICAL SETTING

Just as there are several theories about how adults learn best, there are also several theories about how to teach adults in a clinical setting. The teacher's choice of learning theory and philosophy of teaching will influence the selection of teaching methods. O'Shea (1994) discusses strategies for clinical teaching that compare to the nursing process, including assessment of the learner, determining the learning goals, defining a teaching plan, implementing the plan, and then evaluating the effectiveness of both teaching and learning. She also notes that the clinical practice setting is and cannot be totally predictable as each new patient is an individual with individual needs and wants. However, it is incumbent upon the teacher to focus on the predictable aspects of the clinical setting necessitating knowledge of the setting, the complexity of the patient caseload, the structure and staffing patterns, and support for health professional learners.

Davis, Sawin, and Dunn (1993) in a study of expert nurse practitioner preceptors described a variety of teaching strategies, beginning with orientation to the clinical setting. Introducing the learner to the setting, the staff, and the charting, along with practice guidelines and policies and expectations is a vital first step in teaching in the clinical setting. Use of patient records for review of charting techniques, and discussing the patient mix are other important first steps in clinical teaching. It is helpful for the teacher to talk about their teaching style and to encourage the learner to share their dominant learning style. Pre-conferencing prior to each clinical session is a helpful teaching method to review past learning, agree on learning expectations for the session, and discuss patients to be seen that day. It is beneficial for the teacher to review learner progress to date on specific outcomes, and to clarify any questions or concerns that have been raised by the learner.

Selection of patients to be cared for by the health professional learner helps the teacher control for the complexity of patient needs. For the beginner, the clinical teacher needs to parcel out the patient needs—helping the learner do the history and parts of the physical examination that are less complex and being present to assist as needed. As the learner progresses, more of the patient encounter can be done alone by the learner with the preceptor called when help is needed. Gathering appropriate information (chart review, history-taking, laboratory studies) takes the most time to learn and requires close attention from the teacher. Doing chart reviews together initially is one way of teaching how to do this. Requiring the learner to present the results of the chart review before seeing the patient also gives the teacher the opportunity to affirm positive learning and correct any oversights in the chart review before talking with the patient. Once the learner has demonstrated proficiency in reviewing patient records, the teacher allows the learner to do the chart review and talk with the patient before presenting the case to the preceptor. Eventually, the learner will proceed to the level of complete care before reporting to the preceptor who then verifies the completeness of the care given with both the learner and the patient before the patient leaves the setting.

Role modeling (the learner observing the teacher provide care initially) (Wiseman, 1994), involving the learner in joint patient counseling (letting learner do as much as possible and filling in gaps), and using directed, guided questioning are common teaching methods used in the clinical setting. Post-conferences are another important teaching method. These offer time to encourage reflection on performance, learner self-evaluation, and verification of learner progress. Learners can be asked to briefly present each patient seen that session, or offer a summary of what was done well and areas needing further attention in future sessions. Charting can be reviewed with the learner, noting that good charting reflects clear thinking, just as an orderly, concise yet complete report to the teacher or consultant reflects a similar pattern of clear thinking and good decision-making.

Socratic questioning is most helpful in encouraging critical thinking, thoughtful reflection, and reevaluation of learner decisions in patient care. It is important that such questioning be used to both direct the learning in the novice and to expand the learner's thinking as s/he advances to a level of competence and proficiency. Socratic questioning helps the learner realize how much s/he already knows (reinforces successful prior learning) and how to apply that knowledge to a variety of patient care situations.

Teaching methods for psychomotor skills include demonstration with return demonstration, and practice on models or simulators in a laboratory setting (Johnson, Zerwic, & Theis, 1999), and actual performance of such skills during the care of patients (Wheeler, 1994). It is a given that suturing a placenta for practice is much different that suturing an episiotomy, yet the technique for suturing can be learned before it is needed in clinical practice. As with any skill, repetition improves performance. The challenge of learning skills needed only in emergency situations (manual removal of placenta, intubation, etc.) is that they are infrequent occurrences and therefore require simulation periodically to maintain the skill. Use of mannequins, plastic models, or simulators can help maintain learner readiness to use the skill if an emergency arises.

SUMMARY

Clinical teaching is a wonderful opportunity to share one's enthusiasm for advanced practice nursing and midwifery. In the best of all possible worlds, all those who teach health professional learners should be expert clinicians themselves. At the very least, clinical teachers must be able to practice competently though not at the expert level. The best match of clinical teacher to learner is a placement of the advanced learner with the expert clinician-teacher who has the widest scope of practice allowing the greatest latitude in the learner's performance within safe limits. The less expert clinical teacher will have a limited boundary of safe practice beyond which the learner cannot be allowed to go. This limited boundary is acceptable for the novice learner who needs more direction and structure as they begin their transition from nurse to nurse practitioner or midwife. Teaching in the clinical setting requires knowledge of how people learn, the progression of learning from acquisition to transfer and internalization of behaviors, and methods that assist the learner to take on the role of advanced practice nurse or midwife. Satisfaction comes with each new generation of health professionals that provide health and illness services of highest quality and effectiveness.

REFLECTIONS

Reflect on how your dedication to patient care may either enhance or detract from your ability to allow learners to provide that care. What is your dominant style of teaching and what styles would you like to learn?

REFERENCES

Benner, P. (1984). *From novice to expert: Excellence and power in clinical nurse practice.* Menlo Park, CA: Addison Wesley.

Bevis, E. O. (1978). *Curriculum building in nursing: A process* (2nd ed.). St. Louis: C.V. Mosby.

Blanchard, K. (1985). *Situational leadership II.* Escondido, CA: Blanchard Training and Development Corporation.

Bowling, J. R. (1993). Clinical teaching in the ambulatory care setting: How to capture the teachable moment. *Journal of the American Osteopathic Association, 93*(2), 235–239.

Davis, M., Sawin, K., & Dunn, M. (1993). Teaching strategies used by expert nurse practitioners preceptors: A qualitative study. *Journal of the American Academy of Nurse Practitioners, 5*(1), 27–33.

Evans, B. C. (2000). Clinical teaching strategies for a caring curriculum. *Nursing and Health Care Perspectives, 21*(3), 133–138.

Gaberson, K. B., & Oermann, M. H. (1999). *Clinical teaching strategies in nursing.* New York: Springer Publishing.

Hayes, E. (1994). Helping preceptors mentor the next generation of nurse practitioners. *Nurse Practitioner, 19*(6), 662–666.

Herrmann, M. M. (1997). The relationship between graduate preparation and clinical teaching in nursing. *Journal of Nursing Education, 36*(7), 317–322.

Highet, G. H. (1950). *The art of teaching.* New York: Vintage Books.

Irby, D. M., Ramsey, P. G., Gillmore, G. M., & Schaad, D. (1991). Characteristics of effective clinical teachings of ambulatory care medicine. *Academic Medicine, 66*(1), 54–55.

Johnson, J. H., Zerwigh, J. J., & Theis, S. L. (1999). Clinical simulation laboratory: An adjunct to clinical teaching. *Nurse Educator, 24*(5), 37–41.

Knowles, M. (1970). *The modern practice of adult education: Andragogy vs. pedagogy.* New York: Association Press.

Massarweh, L. J. (1999). Promoting a positive clinical experience. *Nurse Educator, 24*(3), 44–47.

Mosston, M. (1972). *Teaching: From command to discovery.* Somerville, NJ: Wadsworth Publishing Company.

O'Shea, H. S. (1994). Clinical preceptorships: Strategies to enhance teaching and learning. *Journal of Wound, Ostomy and Continence Nursing, 21*(3), 98–105.

O'Shea, H. S., & Parsons, M. (1979). Clinical instruction: Effective and ineffective teacher behaviors. *Nursing Outlook, 26,* 411–415.

Paterson, B. L. (1997). The negotiated order of clinical teaching. *Journal of Nursing Education, 36*(5), 197–205.

Reilly, D. E., & Oermann, M. H. (1992). *Clinical teaching in nursing education.* New York: National League for Nursing (pub. No. 15-2471).

Rideout, E. M. (1994). Letting go: Rationale and strategies for student-centered approaches to clinical teaching. *Nurse Education Today, 14,* 146–151.

Snyder, D. J., & Bunkers, S. J. (1994). Facilitators and barriers for minority students in masters' nursing programs. *Journal of Professional Nursing, 10*(3), 140–146.

Stevens, K. R. (1995). Teaching vision and passion. *Journal of Nursing Education, 34*(3), 99.

Thompson, J. B. (1983). Selected principles of teaching and learning applied to nurse-midwifery clinical education. *Journal of Nurse-Midwifery, 28*(1), 21–29.

Wheeler, L. (1994). Teaching strategies for preceptors of beginning intrapartal students. *Journal of Nurse-Midwifery, 39*(5), 321–325.

Wiseman, R. F. (1994). Role model behaviors in the clinical setting. *Journal of Nursing Education, 33*(9), 404.

CHAPTER 11

Assessment Strategies for Clinical Performance

The real concern in learning and teaching is whether changes are taking place in the behavior of the learner. Any single set of observations can say very little about change. Multiple observations are required to make an adequate assessment about change.

—V. C. Conley,
Curriculum and Instruction in Nursing

SUGGESTED OUTCOMES FOR THIS CHAPTER

At the completion of this chapter the reader will be able to

1. distinguish formative and summative clinical assessment, and
2. identify a variety of clinical assessment tools.

INTRODUCTION

A major goal of the theoretical education in advanced practice nursing and midwifery is to provide a foundation for competent practice. The fundamental reason for developing a body of knowledge in nursing is for the purpose of creating expert nursing practice (Chinn & Kramer, 1999). This is equally true for midwifery. To maintain this holistic approach it is essential that the learner outcomes for theory and practice, developed for the program and for individual courses, are developed concurrently. The curriculum design will determine the specific placement of learning experiences necessary to attain the practice outcomes. It is the role of the educational program to ascertain that at the completion of the program the candidate seeking certification is a knowledgeable, competent, caring, and safe practitioner. This chapter will focus on assessment of the learner in the clinical setting, or *performance assessment*.

Performance assessment is probably one of the most anxiety producing situations for the beginning learner and beginning teacher. Is this anxiety well founded? The authors of this text are of the opinion that this anxiety can be greatly minimized by promoting a conducive teaching-learning environment—one in which the adult learner's past experience is acknowledged and respected, guidance is provided in a constructive framework, and competent and caring role models are available to the learner.

PERFORMANCE OUTCOMES

Objective criteria are essential for appropriate performance assessment. The American College of Nurse-Midwives' (ACNM) standards of practice and core competencies are guidelines for nurse-midwifery and midwifery practice (ACNM, 1997; 1999). Each of the nurse practitioner specialty organizations has documented curriculum guidelines for the specific specialty as well as practice standards (National League for Nursing Accrediting Commission [NLNAC], 1999). As explained in chapter 7, the expected clinical competency outcomes are clearly stated in the program outcomes and with more specificity in the course outcomes. These statements will serve as the basis for performance assessment. It is acknowledged by many teachers that the cognitive and psychomotor domains are incorporated into assessment tools quite readily. The element frequently overlooked is the affective domain, a domain that requires equal attention when using any advanced practice nursing or midwifery assessment tool.

Outcome statements for performance assessment have essentially the same principles as those stated in the competency outcome statements in chapter 7. The outcome is learner centered, observable, stated in very clear terminology without ambiguity, includes the critical elements to determine safe, caring and competent practice, and is based on the accepted standard policy and procedures of the specialty area. Expected outcomes are also determined in relation to the level of the learner.

Advanced practice builds on the knowledge and practice of the professional nurse. Important questions to ask are, "What knowledge, skill, and attitude should be demonstrated or inferred in order to meet the outcome at the advanced practice level? Are these included in the outcome statements?" A first semester or first level practice outcome criteria are based on criteria appropriate for the beginning advanced practitioner. The criteria must be well known and understood by the learner. Of equal importance is that all teachers and/or clinical staff involved in the assessment have similar understanding of what demonstrates competence at each level. Irrespective of the level, it is critical that in the development of practice-stated outcomes there is a clear delineation of the proficiency for each level of learner. The competency in the basic theoretical knowledge would not change with the level of student. However, the expectation for application in practice will differ considerably from a beginning learner in the clinical environment to the learner with repeated opportunities for practice. Another variable is the situation in which this knowledge is integrated. With progression in the program the learner will be expected to move from the normal clinical nursing or midwifery situation to those of more complexity. The stated outcomes used as the basis for the performance assessment must reflect this changing expectation. Irrespective of the level of the learner the underlying criteria for all performance assessment is safety.

FORMATIVE AND SUMMATIVE ASSESSMENT

The formative assessment is a critical component in the attainment of performance competency. The expectation of the teacher during the formative assessment must be in correlation with the level of the learner. During this period, particularly in the case of interpreting client manifestations and beginning advanced manual skills, the learner needs guidance and support. The learning environment should be one of open dialogue, fostering inquiry and critical thinking. A nonthreatening environment promotes optimal clinical learning and decreases learner anxiety. Competencies in the affective area cut across all levels and, if indicated, need open discussion whenever deviations are detected. These areas (discussed in chapter 4) include sensitivity and respect for diversity, including differences related to age, gender, culture, race-ethnicity, socioeconomic status, and ability. Communication patterns with peers, clients, families, and the multidisciplinary team are also important areas for dialogue in the assessment. The formative assessment focuses on the observed strengths in each of the learning domains as well as areas in need of assistance or improvement. The assessment must be authentic, and provide feedback and opportunities to gain additional experience if improvement is indicated. Formative assessment can also inform the teacher of what changes may need to be made in instruction for better understanding and integration of knowledge and skills. Learning plans and performance contracts used in the formative period are discussed in chapter 12.

The summative assessment takes place at a time determined by the program policies or, if indicated for special reasons, at an agreed point in time. A variety of assessment techniques and methods are available. The choice is selected in relation to the goal of the outcome. Strategies to assist each learner to attain the goal of becoming a knowledgeable, competent, and safe practitioner are discussed in chapter 4. Failure to reach the designated clinical competency required in the summative assessment, irrespective of the demonstrated theoretical excellence, can lead to withdrawal from the program. Withdrawal is the least desirable outcome for any performance assessment and all efforts will have been made to assist the learner, including the performance contract discussed in chapter 12, to meet the program or course outcomes.

Assessment Tools

Professional judgment is the foundation for assessment (Brualdi, 1998). This judgment is manifested in observation as well as in the development and use of tools to assist in an objective assessment. It is well recognized that assessment influences learner motivation and learning. An important decision that must be made, as part of curriculum design, is where the knowledge, skill or attitude, and values will be demonstrated. Is it necessary to validate a particular advanced technical skill in a clinical setting? Or can the technical competence be attained in a simulated resource center? What are the key points you want to assess during the application of the skill in the clinical setting? Does the tool you are using focus on technicalities of a procedure, or on a decision-making process while using the skill, or on aspects in the affective domain that can only be observed in the clinical setting? You must ask yourself: Does the assessment tool I am developing or selecting adequately assess the outcome it is meant to assess? Does this outcome require a different or an additional tool in order to have a valid assessment?

Rating Scales

Rating scales can be limited to a quality or frequency judgment, for example: excellent, good, average, fair, or always, frequently, sometimes, never. The quality judgment is open to the individual interpretation of the rater and can result in lack of inter-rater uniformity. This can be overcome, to a degree, by giving explicit criteria for each quality characteristic. The frequency rating scale is very limited in its usefulness as it is documenting a very limited sample that has been observed and omits the many unobserved incidents. Neither rating scale provides the learner with any feedback on strengths or weaknesses.

The quality or frequency scale can also be associated with a number and a descriptive rubric. For example:

Circle the appropriate number to indicate the degree to which the beginning APN learner meets the criteria for presentation of a chart review.

1. Unorganized and does not follow a consistent pattern.
2. Omits significant social problems or laboratory results.
3. Follows a logical order and neglects not more than one significant factor.
4. Follows a logical order and includes all significant factors.

A descriptive rating scale is useful to show progress toward specific outcomes. For example:

Indicate your rating by placing an X along the horizontal line.
1. To what extent does the midwifery learner obtain an organized complete antenatal history on the first visit of a primigravida client?

unorganized approach and incomplete data	gathered and organized data with preceptor guidance	gathered and organized data in a timely fashion independently

Comments:

Checklist

A checklist requires no judgment but simply indicates whether a specific characteristic is present or absent or if a particular action was taken or not taken. In the case of the advanced practice nurse or midwifery learner this can be useful for a performance skill in a simulated situation where the skill is learned and practiced. It has limited value in the clinical area, as many parameters beyond the skill will be assessed simultaneously.

Anecdotal Record

The anecdotal record is a factual description of what is observed. The record is made of positive and negative behavioral incidents. This is a nonjudgmental and objective tool that is extremely valuable for observation or documentation of a specific behavior. It requires a brief and concise description of what the learner said or did, includes only the details that are relevant to the incident, and does not include any interpretation of the incident. Documentation should be made as soon as possible after the observation. The observer's interpretation is documented as a separate notation. This is a useful tool when working with a learner who is being counseled on manifestations of bias, lack of sensitivity, or unsafe practice. A judgment should not be made on a single incident. The observation is shared with the learner and assistance given to alter the behavior. It is important to document the positive incidents that result from the dialogue as well as any repeated negative behavior. If repeated behavior is of a nature to place the student in jeopardy, the documentation becomes a part of the permanent student record. Important points for anecdotal recording are the following: 1) it should be significant, 2) it must be observed accurately, and 3) it must be described precisely and objectively.

The writing of anecdotal records is a skill. The skill can be developed by selecting significant positive behaviors observed and writing an anecdotal record for your own development of the skill until you feel you have reached the point of briefness, conciseness, and accuracy that would convey a true description of the behavior to a non-observer.

Assessment Based on Clinical Objectives

Assessment of learning is a joint responsibility of the learner and teacher. An evaluation tool based on specific clinical objectives is the assessment of choice for the authors. It is most useful to monitor learner progress and provide an opportunity for the adult learner to direct her or his own learning needs. As a formalized tool it can be used by the learner as an ongoing indication of progress and by the preceptor and teacher as an ongoing and summative assessment tool. This combined with specific nursing and midwifery activities, identified for observation by the preceptor or teacher, can validate the learner's ability to meet the clinical objectives.

Videotaping

Videotaping has already been discussed as a teaching-learning strategy. This is also an excellent assessment tool. With the client's permission and the knowledge of the student that this is part of a formal assessment it can serve a dual purpose—formative feedback and assessment.

Seminars

The knowledge base for clinical practice can be assessed very productively through observation of the leaders and participants in seminars—again, with specific objectives for the areas to be assessed and the knowledge of the learners that this is one of the means of assessing clinical knowledge and that it can be part of a formative or summative assessment.

Self-Assessment

Self-assessment can be used in a variety of situations. Following a learning experience that includes an oral clinical presentation the learner can be requested to present a self-assessment at the conclusion of the presentation. There is a tendency for some learners to focus on negative aspects of the work they have presented. It is the role of the teacher to redirect the learner so s/he becomes as comfortable speaking of the positive aspects as of the negative aspects. If extensive feedback is required this should be done privately with the learner.

Maintaining a journal or log focusing on the clinical experiences, that is shared with the teacher at designated intervals, also provides an opportunity for the learner to gauge his/her progress in all domains of learning. Time should be taken by the teacher to explain the purpose and expectations for the journal or log as well as time given to the learner to dialogue about the documented professional growth.

Peer Review

As a member of a profession there is an obligation to participate in a peer review of practice. With specific guidelines this is an excellent opportunity for the advanced practice learner to gain practice in this skill and receive constructive feedback from peers in relation to his or her own progress in practice. This contributes to the formative assessment of the learner.

SUMMARY

There is no one single tool for clinical assessment of the advance practice nurse or midwife. For a valid assessment, a combination of methods and techniques should be used. The most important point is that whichever assessment tool is used, it must be based on the clinical objectives of the course or program. Grading for clinical practice is a moot point for the authors. An advanced practitioner must be a safe and competent practitioner. There is no room for an almost safe or almost competent practitioner. Each practitioner must demonstrate competency in all required areas of practice.

REFLECTIONS

Take yourself back in time to grammar school and high school. Do you recall doing any self-assessment on your academic progress? What were your anxieties? Reflect on your professional preparation. Were you comfortable with clinical assessments? What were your most anxiety producing situations? What assistance did you receive to reduce anxiety? What did you find helpful? What strategies would you now use to assist learners to avoid or reduce anxiety?

REFERENCES

American College of Nurse-Midwives. (1997). *Core competencies for basic midwifery practice.* Washington, DC: Author.

American College of Nurse-Midwives. (1999). *DOA criteria for accreditation of nurse-midwifery and midwifery education programs.* Washington, DC: Author.

Brualdi, A. (1998). *Implementing performance assessment in the classroom. Practical assessment, research and evaluation.* [On-line]. Available: http://ericae.net/pare/getvn.asp?v=6&n=2

Chinn, P., & Kramer, M. (1999). *Theory and nursing: Integrated knowledge development* (5th ed.). St. Louis: Mosby.

Conley, V. C. (1973). *Curriculum and instruction in nursing.* Boston: Little, Brown and Company.

National League for Nursing Accrediting Commission. (1999). Accreditation, standards and criteria for academic quality of post secondary and higher degree programs in nursing [Online]. Available: http://www.accrediting-comm-nlnac.org/

CHAPTER 12

Common Learning Difficulties and Interventions

I've learned that encouragement from a good teacher can turn a student's life around. I've learned that the best way to attend to any problem is to hurry slowly. I've learned that people can change, so give them a chance.

—H. J. Brown,
Live and Learn and Pass It On

SUGGESTED OUTCOMES FOR THIS CHAPTER

At the end of this chapter, the reader will be able to

1. identify and describe common learning difficulties of nurse practitioner and midwifery learners by knowledge domain;
2. define content and appropriate use/timing of learning plans and performance contracts with learners in the clinical setting; and
3. describe teaching strategies that clarify and address specific learning difficulties in the cognitive, affective, and psychomotor domains.

INTRODUCTION

When one is learning a new role, task, or way of interacting with others, there will always be moments when the learning button is put on pause. That pause may be an opportunity to reflect on what is going on, a challenge to identify and move beyond perceived barriers to learning, or a normal plateau in the learning curve where practice is needed to reinforce that the learner can be successful and therefore take new risks in learning. What both teacher and learner hope is that the pause button will not remain on permanently so that all learning stops.

As teachers, we understand and know that people learn in different ways and at different rates. As teachers in a clinical discipline, we are also acutely aware of the need to provide safe care to patients that, in turn, requires the learner to acquire knowledge and apply it to clinical care in a relatively short period of time (Reilly & Oermann, 1992). The time frame for learning in an advanced practice nursing or midwifery program is based on faculty experience, curriculum design, expected competencies and outcomes, and university course and semester guidelines. The program length is generally designed for the adult learner who is above average intellectually and quick to learn and do. The program length defined by the faculty allows time for learning, time for making mistakes, and a predetermined time when the novice clinician must demonstrate successful clinical practice with a variety of patients. It is a rare APN educational program that allows the adult learner unlimited time to learn, though some of the more nontraditional programs affiliated with universities may have more flexibility in the time frame for a particular course or unit of study. Experienced faculty and clinical teachers develop a keen sense for knowing when learning is not proceeding well, when intervention is needed, and what intervention may be indicated with a particular learning difficulty. Novice teachers need to develop this clinical learning knowledge and intuition so that they can diagnose and intervene in a timely manner.

This chapter is about those times when learning seems to have stopped and what the teacher can do to help overcome barriers to continued learning. It is the responsibility of the teacher to assist the learner in defining the what and why of this pause in learning, and it is the responsibility of the learner to determine how they can proceed in a timely manner, including getting the needed help from others.

COMMON LEARNING DIFFICULTIES AND TEACHING STRATEGIES

The authors have found it helpful to discuss common learning difficulties within APN and basic midwifery learners by knowledge domain. This is done to assist both the novice teacher and learner in defining the learning problem and designing appropriate intervention. It is recognized that more than one knowledge domain can be involved in a learning difficulty, and therefore intervention needs to be designed to fit all dimensions of the learning problem. Teasing apart the components of a learning problem first and then designing a plan for overcoming each component can be helpful to new teachers. The examples given below are used to illustrate the concept of diagnosis and suggested intervention in the psychomotor, cognitive, and affective domains of learning.

Common Psychomotor Difficulties

The authors have categorized the major learning difficulties in the psychomotor domain in four areas: 1) hands do not work well, 2) hand-eye coordination is lacking, 3) efficiency and speed is lacking at appropriate skill level, and 4) tongue engages before brain engaged. A few examples of such learning difficulties are offered to illustrate each of these areas of psychomotor distress.

Clinicians know the importance of having their hands under control when touching patients or performing a particular skill. No one enjoys several needle sticks to obtain a blood specimen or several attempts in locating the cervix with a vaginal speculum. Trembling hands can lead to patient discomfort as well as learner discomfort. Repeated contamination of a sterile field, knocking over equipment, or overly aggressive touch during a physical examination are signs of a psychomotor problem that needs to be corrected if good patient care is to be the result. The teacher (and often the learner) detects this learning problem through observation—watching the body and hand movements during clinical care.

Reasons for trembling hands or "klutzy" behavior vary. Sometimes the hands tremble when the learner is unsure whether they really know how to do something. If this is the reason, then the appropriate teaching strategy/intervention is to teach how to do it through demonstration, return demonstration, and multiple opportunities for the learner to practice the skills on models or simulators with coaching and encouragement from the teacher (Blanchard, 1985). If the reason for shaking hands is fear of doing something wrong, then the intervention is similar to above but the teacher also needs to help the learner recognize and work through the fear. Reinforcement of positive gains in control of one's body and hands also helps to increase the confidence level of the learner so that the hands shake less. Occasionally the teacher may need to gently place her hands on top of the learner's hands to steady them. This touching must be proceeded by a verbal cue that the teacher is going to do this so that the learner is not surprised nor offended. A surprised touching may cause the learner to drop what she is holding or to withdraw her hands from the patient quickly—just the opposite of what the teacher intends. If the learner has a physiological tremor, this will be obvious early on in the educational program, and the learner often has adopted ways to minimize the tremor during clinical care.

Hand-eye coordination is more of a challenge to some learners than others. This learning difficulty often shows up when the learner moves from the safety of the laboratory setting to the clinical setting where the skill must be performed on patients. One example of lack of hand-eye coordination is wrapping one's fingers around the neck of a newborn head as it emerges from the birth canal without realizing that the grip on the neck is too tight—the eyes see where the hands are but the fingers do not send the message of grip and the need to stay away from the infant's neck. Another example of such behavior is when the teacher observes that the learner's hands are kneading the abdomen of a very pregnant woman rather than using the smooth, purposeful approach learned in the classroom and demonstrated on a model. The learner knows how to perform Leopold's maneuvers, can explain how, but does not interpret what her hands are doing even though she is watching them. The eyes and the hands are not working together. Encouraging the learner to take up knitting, needlepoint, or other fun activities as practice for hand-eye coordination often improves this coordination in the clinical setting. Also, talking about what the teacher is observing and asking the learner to practice the skills and concentrate on what her eyes are telling her about her performance of the skill can be helpful in addressing this psychomotor difficulty.

Efficiency and decreasing the time it takes to perform a particular skill come normally with practice and repeated exposure to performing such a skill. Though the teacher nor learner cannot expect "perfect" performance of a skill (timely, efficient, accurate results) on the first or second try, there is a time when the learner must perform in this way. It is common to be slow in skill performance to begin with, and to decrease one's time of performance as the learner becomes both competent and confident in performing the skill. If the learner cannot perform a complete history and physical examination on a relatively healthy person within 45 minutes by the end of an educational program, s/he will be of questionable use in practice—especially in today's managed cost environments that limit provider time with patients in the interests of increasing patient volume and revenue.

One of the authors developed an approach to teaching efficiency and speed in the repair of episiotomy or laceration with novice midwifery students. She set the total time limit of repair at 20 minutes, and allowed the novice practitioner the first 15 minutes to sew. At the end of 15 minutes, the teacher finished whatever was left of the repair, making sure the woman was not required to remain in an uncomfortable position longer than 20 minutes. At first, the teacher guided the midwifery learner in repairing the vaginal layer (begin with easiest and reinforce positive learning). During the second try, the teacher encouraged the learner to spend the time on repairing the perineum. When all aspects of repair were performed correctly (with positive reinforcement) by the learner, she was encouraged to work on speed as she put all of them together in 15–20 minutes. This approach to teaching the skill reinforced the woman's comfort and reassured the learner that they would have experience with all aspects of sewing before being required to sew a laceration or episiotomy completely. If the learner was not progressing in time and efficiency, she was asked to practice her sewing daily on placentas, chicken breasts or whatever medium was available for practice. Ofttimes the combination of practice with reinforcement of correct technique along with re-peated opportunities to work with an actual patient within a short time frame supported the learner in picking up both speed and efficiency. The teacher was also known to whisper in the learner's ear a gentle reminder of, "Pretend you are in a hurry!" The combination of teacher physical presence, support, and humor resulted in successful learning.

Tongue engaging before brain can be a personality trait or common practice that was never called into question before, or it can result from anxiety or lack of knowledge without realizing it. Learner styles are quite different, but in patient encounters it is important to think before talking or doing. Sometimes the teacher only needs to remind the learner to think before talking, and the problem is solved. At other times, the teacher will need to spend time in post-conference to help the learner become more aware of what she is saying and doing. Use of videotaping with patient consent allows the learner an opportunity to see themselves as viewed by both the patient and teacher. This often helps the learner understand what is being said about their performance and recognize the need to change—a first step in changing any behavior. Anxiety pushes some individuals to talk a lot, while others become very quiet. Helping the learner identify the source of anxiety and then addressing it can help the learner overcome this learning difficulty. If the reason a learner is speaking out before thinking through what she is saying is because she thinks she "knows it all" without realizing her knowledge deficits, careful reflection on possible areas needing more information can be helpful. If the learner is acting before thinking because she thinks if she talks a lot, the teacher or patient will not realize she doesn't know the answer, the teacher intervention now becomes focused on helping the learner admit what she does not know instead of making things up, and then supporting and coaching her to fill her knowledge gap.

Cognitive Learning Difficulties

As with the previous section, the author has found it helpful to categorize cognitive learning problems as follows: 1) brain works independently of hands/eyes; 2) critical thinking is lacking or inconsistent; 3) theory base is incomplete, marginal, or not being used; and 4) communication skills with clients, faculty, or peers are inappropriate. One can note the interface of psychomotor and cognitive in these categories, though the dominant learning difficulty is in the cognitive domain.

Brain Independent of Hands/Eyes

One example of the brain working independently of the hands/eyes that can be quickly identified by the teacher is when the teacher asks the learner what s/he is doing and the learner describes correctly what should be done while doing something else. While working with hundreds of midwifery learners, the author observed a pattern of novice learner behavior she describes as "elbow dyslexia." During the first few births, the learner will often be able to describe where the hands should be placed for the birth, can talk herself through the birth, can watch her own performance, and still not be able to explain how the baby ended up in her arms. It is almost as if something has interrupted the flow of information from the brain to the hands and vice versa—the brain knows what to do, the hands are doing something, but the brain cannot explain what the hands have just done. The primary reason for the interruption in the flow of information is anxiety and genuine awe at attending those first few births as a midwife. Another example of lack of coordination between the brain (knowledge) and performance (behavior/action) is when the learner can tell you what s/he plans to do and why, and then proceeds to do something else that is inappropriate for the patient. The teacher works with the learner to determine why this is happening, and whether the intervention should be further study, clinical simulation (Johnson, Zerwic, & Theis, 1999), or more exposure to a variety of patients with a variety of needs.

Critical Thinking Inconsistent

Lack of ability to think critically or inconsistent use of critical thinking in the care of patients is a serious cognitive learning problem. It is usually apparent in the following aspects of clinical care:

1. Data collection incomplete or unorganized
2. Decisions are inaccurate, based on incomplete data
3. Learner unable to define appropriate role in clinical situation
4. Plan of care incomplete, inaccurate, does not involve patient or consider alternatives
5. Caregiving unsafe, inappropriate, incomplete
6. Learner unable or unwilling to evaluate self or plan of care

Intervention needed will depend on which area of critical thinking is lacking. For example, if data collection is disorganized, practice with many charts ahead of the office session can improve the learner's ability to review a chart in an orderly and complete manner. An unorganized approach to gathering information from the patient can be overcome by using audiotapes of history taking (with permission of patient) and having the learner listen to these to hear themselves and to work on organizing their approach to history taking. Unsafe clinical practice requires an immediate intervention from the clinical teacher to protect the patient. Depending on the severity of the safety infraction, the learner may not be allowed to continue in the clinical setting until remediation has been completed, or may be asked to leave the program. Inability to accurately evaluate one's performance in the clinical setting requires immediate attention as well. The teacher may note that the learner either overestimates his or her own abilities, or constantly demeans their own performance (hypercritical). The former situation is a teacher's worst nightmare because the teacher can no longer trust that the learner knows their limits of practice and therefore, can become a danger to patient welfare. This situation requires very close supervision and often means that the level of independent practice required for graduation may not be met (see performance contract section that follows). On the other hand, the learner who has a tendency to be hypercritical and focuses primarily on what they missed, did wrong, or don't know, offers the teacher a different and more positive challenge in promoting critical thinking. At the very least, the teacher is reassured that the learner will not try anything they don't know how to do. However, this learner may also not take the risks to try new approaches to care without the teacher present, limiting autonomous decision-making. Reinforcement of positive learning, things done well, and encouragement often help the hypercritical learner to relax and continue learning. Both situations must be overcome if competent, responsible clinicians are to result.

Theory Base Marginal or Incomplete

One of the easiest ways to determine whether the learner has adequately prepared for the clinical experience is to question their knowledge base. In the clinical setting, this often takes the form of asking the learner why they did what they did, or what they plan to do. Seeking and sharing rationale for clinical practice is invaluable in expanding the knowledge base of novice learners. However, it is most appropriate to expect that the learner come to the clinical setting with a baseline knowledge and be willing to learn what is needed to care for the patients in that setting. This means that the faculty of the educational program, if different from the clinical teacher, need to make sure the clinical teacher knows the level of student assigned and the expected knowledge base. If the learner can respond correctly to questions of why s/he plans a particular course of action but then does not carry this out, the teacher needs to help the learner to find out the reasons they are not using their knowledge base. Sloppiness is unacceptable in patient care and often suggests that the learner does not like the patients they are taking care of (discrimination). Immediate intervention by the teacher is needed, along with exploration of value biases.

Inappropriate Communication Skills

Some might wonder why communication skills are included in the cognitive domain and affective domain rather than in the psychomotor, but here we are talking about communication on the basis of knowledge, critical thinking, and relationships (also affective). Experienced teachers often note that what comes out of the mouth of learners is a reflection of how they think. If the clinical teacher listens closely to a learner report on a patient encounter, the organization of that report along with the content will reveal much about the learner's thinking patterns as well as knowledge base that informs action or choices. The manner in which a learner talks with patients is very reflective of both cognitive and affective domains of learning. Once again the learner's value biases can be picked up and need to be addressed in the privacy of a teacher-learner conference. Asking the learner to review the code of ethics (American College of Nurse-Midwives, 1993; American Medical Association, 1985; American Nurses Association, 1976; International Council of Nurses, 2000) for their professional role and analyze the expected moral behavior toward patients can be a most helpful learning exercise. If the learner tells the patient incorrect information, the teacher needs to intervene at the moment to correct the information, but can do so in a nonthreatening manner and then approach the learner afterward to discuss why they said what they said. Intervention will be based on whether the inappropriate communication is result of gaps in knowledge, unconscious value biases, or engaging one's tongue before putting the brain in gear—all of which were discussed above.

Affective Learning Difficulties

Affective learning problems can be grouped together under the following headings: 1) unwilling to make a decision even though learner has adequate knowledge base, 2) unwilling to assume accountability for actions/care, 3) refusal to include patient and family in care discussions and decisions (lack of informed consent), 4) lack of integrity—dishonest with patients and faculty, and 5) lack of common sense—always seeking out zebras instead of the common or ordinary (cows). Some examples of these affective learning problems follow with suggested teacher interventions.

The learner who consistently demonstrates an unwillingness to make decisions or assume responsibility for his or her actions is often afraid. These are the learners with limited life experience or limited nursing practice, and therefore the practice of nursing is new to them along with learning the advanced practice role. On the other hand, experienced nurses who return for graduate study in an advanced practice or midwifery role may also be afraid of this new role because they are not used to the buck stopping with them (could often defer to doctor's orders or direction rather than giving the order themselves). Both situations require teacher support, discussion, and direction for the novice learner to take the risk of making the decision, to use their knowledge, and to be responsible for their choices. Adult learners have many years of being responsible for their personal choices and it is the challenge to the teacher to help the learner see the similarities between personal and patient care choices.

Lack of informed participation and decision-making by patients is unethical when one is working with competent adults (Thompson & Thompson, 1985). Sometimes the novice learner is trying to take care of the patient in a paternalistic way, and some patients really enjoy being taken care of when they could really do it themselves. However, the goal of promoting health and preventing illness will not be accomplished if patients are not viewed by health professionals as both competent and responsible for their own health. If the learner is deliberately making decisions for the competent patient because s/he thinks s/he knows best, then this approach is clearly unethical, as the patient's right to self-determination is violated (see chapter on ethics and values).

A learner who lacks integrity has no place in the health professions. This is a serious character flaw, and needs to be identified as early as possible in the educational program. In most APN and midwifery programs, evidence of lack of integrity, such as falsifying patient records or lying about what was or was not done for a patient are grounds for immediate expulsion. Fortunately, lack of integrity is a rare find in graduate education in nursing, though the authors have had experience with such learners in their teaching careers. There may be a hint of dishonesty in a learner who is not comfortable admitting to the teacher when they do not know. Setting a tone of openness at the beginning of the program, and reinforcing the importance of gaining comfort in saying, "I don't know, but I will find out," is a valuable teaching strategy. When a learner hears the teacher admit they do not know everything and that this is okay as long as one is willing to learn what is missing, they often become more comfortable themselves in admitting to gaps in their learning with a willingness to fill them.

Lack of common sense is another personality characteristic that needs attention if the learner is to proceed to competent clinical practice. The very brightness of APN and midwifery students can lead to an overabundance of theoretical knowledge gained without the ability to sort through what is important and what is probably not going to be useful in daily practice. The clinical teacher needs to balance her support for theoretical knowledge with the practical advice on what to focus on in patient care. Sorting through the extremes to find the commonplace is a joint effort of teacher and learner in the clinical setting. The teacher who remembers how he learned to do this and shares that learning with others can help the novice begin to gain common sense in their approach to patient care.

LEARNING PLANS AND PERFORMANCE CONTRACTS

When learning has stopped longer than expected, it is important for the teacher and learner to sit together and discuss what is going on and how learning can proceed. The authors have found it helpful to use both learning plans (Knowles, 1978) and performance contracts (McHugh & Armstrong, 1991) to address learning difficulties in the clinical area. Each of these tools will be described briefly below. Use of such tools facilitates early diagnosis of learning problems, joint problem-solving, and planning for timely intervention so that learning can continue. These tools also provide a written record of both learner and teacher agreement on the definition of the problem, the suggested strategies for overcoming the difficulty, the performance outcomes expected, and the time frame for formative evaluation of progress and summative evaluation.

The process for diagnosing and treating learning difficulties in the clinical setting involves early diagnosis of the learning problem, agreement of learner and teacher on the nature of the problem, and why it has occurred, so that a plan for overcoming the difficulty is reached that is reasonable, clearly defined, and doable within the time constraints of the educational program. The teacher needs to consider several questions before and during the development of either a learning plan or performance contract:

1. Is it realistic for the learner to overcome the identified deficit within the semester or program time limits?
2. Is the nature of the identified deficit sufficiently serious to warrant an immediate performance contract or will the learning plan be the first step?
3. What are the appropriate considerations to take into account when designing a time frame for either a learning plan or performance contract?
4. Who should be involved in learner conferences (faculty or course coordinator, clinical teacher, learner)?
5. How much allowance should be given for family/personal problems that are interfering with learning the advanced practice nursing or midwifery role?
6. What are the university/program policies on progression of learning and offering services to the learner (psychological counseling and/or testing)?
7. What are the university guidelines on recording learning plans and performance contracts and including them in the learner record?
8. Is the outside time limit for continuing in the program clearly identified, realistic, and understood by all parties?
9. How will one assure that both teacher and learner stick to stated criteria for evaluation of learner progress?
10. If the learner is not successful in overcoming the learning deficit, what action is supported by the program and university?

Learning Plans (Adapted from Knowles, 1978)

By definition, a learning plan is designed by the learner when s/he has noted an area of clinical deficiency early enough so there is time to correct the deficit. Both learner and teacher agree on the description of the learning problem, the steps and resources needed to overcome the deficit, and the time period allowed.

In general, clinical deficiencies that respond best to learning plans do not involve questions of clinical safety. They most commonly involve psychomotor skill development, organization of thinking, and overcoming the fear of making decisions in patient care. Chan and Wai-tong (2000) describe the benefits of using learning plans to increase learner autonomy and motivation for learning. They also found that clinical teacher-learner communication and sharing increased. Specific details of the learning plan are written, kept on file until the outcomes are achieved, and used for interim evaluation of progress. The steps followed in designing a learning plan include

1. Clearly define the learning deficit, including learning needs and direction of expected growth.
2. Identify the resources and strategies to be used to overcome this deficit, including use of practice sessions, number of patient encounters, and extra clinical time.
3. Define the time frame for completion of the learning plan including interim formative evaluation against performance outcomes and the final summative evaluation of achievement.
4. Have the student review his or her learning plan with the course coordinator and solicit input on strategies to promote successful learning.
5. Implement the learning plan and revise and update as needed.
6. Confirm completion of the learning plan in timely manner with all involved.
7. If the learning plan does not overcome deficit, consider a move to a performance contract.

A sample student-designed learning plan might read this way:
Learning Deficiency: Poor visualization and repair of episiotomy.
Satisfactory Performance: Ability to identify layers involved in episiotomy; ability to suture episiotomy with minimal coaching.
Unsatisfactory Performance: Failure to identify layers accurately; failure to repair appropriately.
Steps to Resolution: Practice on foam and placentas, review physiology of perineum, review steps of episiotomy repair, demonstrate technique on placenta or chicken breast.
Learning Resources: Oxorn and Foote, Varney, Fry video.
Date for Review: One week from today (date).
Date for Completion of Plan: Two weeks from today providing exposure to minimum of two episiotomy repairs.

Date: _____

Signatures: _____   _____
                        (Teacher)   (Learner)

Performance Contracts

A performance contract is used when learning has stopped or performance indicates a severe deficit in knowledge and/or skill in relation to performance expected of learner at a given level (McHugh & Armstrong, 1991). A performance contract is appropriate when the identified problem in learning may lead to significant consequences for the learner (e.g., expulsion from the program) or the client (unsafe learner practice). A performance contract may also be used when the learner has been unable to complete a learning plan or when there is disagreement between the learner and the teacher on the nature of the learning deficit. The decision to initiate a performance contract is reached in consultation with the program faculty if different from the clinical teacher.

The content of the performance contract is similar to that of the learning plan, with final consequences of failure to meet the stated performance behaviors leading to failure in the educational program. Once again, this contract is written and signed by both learner and clinical teacher and progress shared with program faculty. If the terms of the contract are not met within the defined time frame, the final action taken is recorded on the contract and becomes a part of the learner's academic record in many institutions.

As a novice teacher, one will immediately understand the importance of identifying learning needs early in the clinical experience. The move to either a learning plan or performance contract can be either positive or negative from the perspective of learner or teacher. For example, learning plans defined and designed by learners are perceived as positive by teachers as they realize the learner knows what they don't know and is willing to learn. Learners sometimes think they are labeled by teachers and classmates if they are on a learning plan, and can be anxious about how their efforts will be perceived. Reassurance of the positive nature of identifying one's own learning needs and then planning ways to meet those needs can be offered by the teacher. Performance contracts are most often seen as negative by the learner, a visible definition that they are in trouble and need immediate help. Teachers also treat performance contracts with more attention than learning plans, for they understand that attaining the specified outcomes is vital to the future career of the learner. It is important for the teacher to be supportive of learners who need either learning plans or performance contracts, for both are tools to enhance learning and contribute to successful clinical practice in novice learners.

SUMMARY

As noted at the beginning of this chapter, all of us will have times in our lives when for a variety of reasons there is a pause in our learning. Quick identification of the reasons we have stopped learning helps us to move forward. Individuals who chose admission to advanced practice nursing or midwifery programs wish to succeed. The great majority will do so, especially if their learning needs are clearly identified and attended to in a timely manner. The teacher can facilitate this success in learning.

REFLECTIONS

Think about a specific situation in which learning seems to have stopped. How did you know that learning had paused or stopped? What did you do? What did the learner do? How was it resolved? What would you do differently, if anything, if a similar situation arose in your clinical teaching?

REFERENCES

American College of Nurse-Midwives. (1993). *Code of ethics for nurse-midwives.* Washington, DC: Author.

American Medical Association. (1985). *Principles of medical ethics.* Chicago: Author.

American Nurses Association. (1976). *Code for nurses.* Washington, DC: Author.

Blanchard, K. (1985). *Situational leadership II: The article* [SL-0018-04]. Escondido, CA: Blanchard Training and Development, Inc.

Brown, H. J. (1992). *Live and learn and pass it on.* Nashville, TN: Rutledge Hill Press.

Chan, S. W., & Wai-tong, C. (2000). Implementing contract learning in a clinical context: A report on a study. *Journal of Advanced Nursing, 31*(2), 298–305.

International Council of Nurses. (2000). *The ICN code of ethics for nurses.* Geneva: Author.

Johnson, J. H., Zerwic, J. J., & Theis, S. L. (1999). Clinical simulation laboratory: An adjunct to clinical teaching. *Nurse Educator, 24*(5), 37–41.

Knowles, M. (1978). *The adult learner: A neglected species* (2nd ed.). Houston: Gulf Publishing Company.

McHugh, M. K., & Armstrong, P. (1991). *Performance contracts.* Hyden, KY: Frontier School of Midwifery and Family Nursing.

Reilly, D. E., & Oermann, M. H. (1992). *Clinical teaching in nursing education.* New York: National League for Nursing.

Thompson, J. E., & Thompson, H. O. (1985). *Bioethical decision making for nurses.* Norwalk, CT: Appleton-Century-Crofts.

CHAPTER 13

Establishing and Maintaining Clinical Sites

Good teaching is supported by strong and visionary leadership, and very tangible institutional support—resources, personnel, and funds.

—R. Leblanc,
"Good Teaching: The Top Ten Requirements"

SUGGESTED OUTCOMES FOR THIS CHAPTER

At the end of this chapter, the reader will be able to

1. determine (define) the administrative details required to establish clinical learning sites for advanced practice nurses and midwives,
2. identify university requirements for contracts with clinical learning sites and how these are negotiated,
3. define the criteria needed for selection of clinical learning sites and preceptors, and
4. describe the preparation of preceptors needed for clinical supervision and teaching.

INTRODUCTION

Good teaching requires not only a well-prepared, dedicated, enthusiastic, and knowledgeable teacher. As noted by LeBlanc (1999) in his description of the top ten requirements of good teaching, good teaching must be supported by visionary leadership and tangible institutional support. Learning in a clinical discipline also requires the vision and strong support of clinical practices and institutions where the role of advanced practice nurse and midwife will be modeled, learned, and internalized as the learner moves from novice to advanced beginner in their chosen career path. This chapter is about the role of teacher and academic units in the establishment and maintenance of sites for clinical learning. The administrative, interpersonal, political, and educational elements of creating a positive learning environment in clinical settings will be presented for direction and reflection as the reader reviews her or his individual role in their academic and clinical settings.

ADMINISTRATIVE DETAILS

Many individuals who elect a formal role as teacher in nursing and midwifery come to that decision following years as a clinician. They are committed to preparing the next generation of APNs and midwives and eager to share their wisdom and insight into professional practice with novice learners. Many new teachers in a clinical specialty, however, are not particularly thrilled or knowledgeable about the administrative effort needed to build and maintain the clinical base for new learners. Yet the teacher and academic unit's success in developing the next generation of highly skilled nurses and midwives is totally dependent on the availability and support of clinical practices. No advanced practice nursing or midwifery program can be successful without strong, high quality clinicians who are willing to share their patients with the academic unit and their learners. It is the bias of the authors that equal attention must be given to the development, nurturing, support, and maintenance of clinical sites and clinical preceptors as is given to the development of the academic program and core faculty. This is a partnership for the future of health and illness care, and all are vital to its success.

The administrative details required to establish clinical learning sites for advanced practice nursing and midwifery learners begin with making contact with a particular site to explore and foster interest among the expert practitioners in that site. Prior to this initial contact, the academic unit will have gathered institutional or practice data related to quality of care and standards of practice as reviewed by an external agency such as JCAHO (Joint Commission on the Accreditation of Healthcare Organizations), National Association of Childbearing Centers (NACC), or evidence of external peer review of the practice. In other words, the academic program needs to know that the potential clinical site/practice and its practitioners comprise an appropriate context for the learner to learn their advanced practice role. Academic faculty need to avoid the temptation to use any available clinical site without checking out the standard of care beforehand. This is especially important when a geographic area becomes saturated with several APN or midwifery programs, and competition increases for clinical sites.

The authors suggest four stages in the development and maintenance of clinical learning sites (Beebe, 1980). These are 1) exploration, 2) preparation, 3) utilization, and 4) ongoing evaluation. Each of these stages will be discussed in some detail.

Stage I: Exploration

There are several steps in exploring potential clinical sites for learning APN or midwifery roles. Initial contact is usually made by telephone following referral of the practice director's name to the academic program. Program faculty learn of new practices in the area through a variety of networks, personal contact, or direct contacts from the practice itself. A personal visit to the site goes a long way in reinforcing the important role such a practice plays in the education of APNs and midwives. Sitting down with the practice director in their environment sets a positive tone of respect and says that one cares enough about the practitioners that the teacher will take the time to physically visit the site. This site visit also affords the opportunity to see the physical setting, meet the various personnel who interact with patients, and note the volume and type of patients who come for health and illness services.

The main goals of this initial or exploratory site visit are to determine the feasibility of assigning learners to the site and discussion of who will be the primary clinical teacher (i.e., whether program faculty will be needed or will practice personnel assume this role). Several established APN and midwifery programs have a clinical site data form that is completed by the practice staff and returned to the academic program (see Appendix E for a sample data sheet). This data sheet includes where the site is located, who the practice staff are, what types and volume of patients are available for the learners, and what specific health requirements must be met for learners to be placed in this setting. The data sheet is maintained on file with the academic program and often kept along with the Agency Contract (see below).

During the exploratory visit, the program representative reviews the practice policies and protocols with the practitioners. Discussion of how these reflect what is taught in the educational program follows and reinforces the adequacy of fit between what the learner is expected to learn and what s/he will see modeled in the practice site. The program representative should also have copies of and review the curricular pattern, philosophy, and content sequence and encourage questions and comments from the practice staff. Often educational programs seek out their graduates for clinical teaching, but should not assume that the graduate is up to date on the current curriculum and expectations. Once the overall program is reviewed and questions addressed, the discussion should turn to details of expectations of both clinical teachers and learners in the clinical setting. Refer to the latter section of this chapter for full discussion of expectations of both teachers and learners in a clinical setting.

The exploratory visit should also result in a decision on the type, level, and number of learners that can be accommodated at a given time in the practice along with the name of the primary contact for any placement issues. A meeting with nursing, medical, and administrative personnel may follow, depending on the structure of the practice and institutional requirements. For example, if a program is exploring the use of a freestanding birth center for placements of midwifery learners, the administrative authority may be the midwifery director of the practice. However, if one is talking with a primary care physician practice affiliated with a larger health system, there may be several administrative persons that need to agree to any affiliation with the academic unit. Before the program representative leaves the clinical site, s/he must know who will receive and process the university contract or letter of agreement (name, title, address). In most instances, the letter of agreement or official contract originates from the university or academic institution, and must be in place before the first learner enters the facility.

Final aspects of the site visit may include discussion of payment, whether in dollars or in kind, for the teaching, supervision, and evaluation of learners. Most APN and midwifery programs do not have extra dollars to pay for clinical teaching; however, payment in kind is usually quite acceptable to the clinicians. Examples of payment in kind include joint appointments of key clinicians, and continuing education opportunities including specific clinical updates in the setting itself, library privileges, or special certificates of appreciation. Specific details about learner housing, costs, transportation, and equipment needs such as cell phones or pagers are also discussed and noted. The program representative confirms the legal requirements for licensure of the APN or midwifery student and whether a copy of the nursing license is needed in the institution. Evidence of liability coverage by the academic unit/learner is often needed by the practice site, including limits of liability. Some midwifery sites require evidence of $1–$3 million insurance coverage as a minimum. Details of limits of liability are often described in the Agency Agreement as discussed below.

As the program representative and practice personnel complete their discussion, a preliminary decision is made as to whether this clinical practice will become a learning environment for students. This moves the development process into the second stage of development.

Stage II: Preparation

The preparation stage for confirming a clinical site/practice for APN and midwifery learners begins at the university with the initiation of the contract or letter of agreement. Each academic unit will have its own process for health agency agreements, and faculty need to pay attention to all the details in finalizing such an agreement. Time must be adequate to obtain needed university and agency signatures before the learner can actually be in the clinical environment. The very nature of advanced practice nursing and midwifery education on the graduate level means that the great majority of learners will already be licensed nurses. Direct entry midwifery programs need to arrange for the special requirements and needs of their non-nurse learners in the practice site as licensure is not an option.

Selection of the specific learners to be assigned to a particular practice site begins within the program faculty group. Criteria such as level of learner matched to complexity of patient caseload, geographic match between learner and site, or type of experience matched with specific learner needs are reviewed when making these assignments. Some program faculty encourage their learners to identify potential practice sites and other programs insist that learners not approach practices—the program makes the selection of student assignments and sites. It is not uncommon for practitioners to request only "the best and the brightest" learners be assigned to them, especially in a busy practice where minimal time is available for teaching. The program faculty, however, need to gently reinforce the need for teaching time, the possible assignment of one practitioner as primary preceptor, or the addition of a program clinical teacher into the practice to assure that the learner has the support and supervision needed to guide their development as APNs or midwives.

The necessary documents needed by the practice site need to be collated at the program and sent as a package to the site. Programs need to establish an organized database of learner information so that the learner is not constantly asked to give copies or evidence of immunizations, nursing licensure, etc. It is important to advise the learner well in advance of the need for a state nursing license in states used for clinical learning that are outside the home state of the educational program. It may take several months to obtain this license, so many programs that routinely use several contiguous states for clinical learning make sure the applicants know of this need before they are matriculated into the program. A summary of commonly requested documents on learners to be assigned to a given practice site include 1) verification of immunization status including Hepatitis C, 2) proof of malpractice coverage (usually done through the university), 3) proof of nursing licensure in state, 4) brief resume, 5) learning profile, and 6) summary of learner performance to date. As noted earlier, the actual documents will vary from program to program and site to site, but the importance of making sure these are complete and provided in a timely manner to the practice site is crucial to maintaining the site.

Once the program site coordinator is designated in the academic unit, that person returns to the practice site to tour the facilities, observe the staff, and communicate with all those who will have contact with the learners. The site coordinator paves the way for the introduction of new learners for the first time or reinforces past successes of the site in preparing competent clinicians. Questions and concerns are addressed, and recognition given to the importance of this site to the educational program as well as to the health of the people served by the site. The final orientation of clinicians to the program curriculum and clinical evaluation tools is provided during this visit, along with confirmation of details of assignment patterns (days of week, hours per session, clinical area). The site coordinator may also review the strengths and needs of the assigned learners along with expected performance outcomes at the end of the assigned time.

If the site practitioners are to be the clinical teachers, an orientation to this role should be given before the first learners are assigned. Refer to the section later in this chapter on the preparation of preceptors. The site coordinator establishes a mutually agreed upon time for communication with the practice staff. For the first level learner, it is best to communicate on a weekly or biweekly basis via telephone to assure progress in learning and early identification of learning difficulties. For the advanced level learner, biweekly to monthly contact may be established. In most APN and midwifery programs, program teachers meet with learners every 2 weeks to review progress in meeting performance outcomes and to discuss how things are going in the clinical site. Standardized forms for reporting from clinical teacher to program faculty or course coordinators facilitate these periodic telephone conversations, and help focus the evaluation strategies of importance in learning the APN or midwifery practice role (see Appendix F for sample report form). It is vital for the program site coordinator to reinforce that s/he is available at any time should an emergency learning problem arise, and that the clinical site teaching staff are never alone in determining the progress of learning—it is a shared endeavor.

One of the final steps in the preparation phase is making sure the assigned learner makes contact with the practice staff before appearing in the site. This allows the opportunity to set up a face-to-face meeting with the clinical teachers/ preceptors and a time for orientation to the site and its specific requirements such as record keeping, review of policies and procedures, and other expectations of practitioners before the learner begins seeing patients. The learner also should share their specific learning needs, strengths, and expected outcomes with the practice staff and discuss what is realistically possible given the nature of the practice, caseload mix, and volume of patients. Learners, program faculty, and practice personnel need to be united in purpose and enthusiasm for learning. Ongoing communication and sharing of successes as well as problems in an atmosphere of trust, mutual respect, and enthusiasm for learning and quality patient care can sustain the clinical learning environment for many years.

Stage III: Utilization

Once the APN or midwifery learner is functioning in the clinical setting, it is important to maintain the contact between program and practice personnel. A suggested protocol to be used during these set times for telephone contact includes comments on 1) the learner's adjustment to the clinical setting, 2) experiences to date, 3) learner progress in meeting performance outcomes, 4) compatibility of learner with practice staff and setting, 5) progress in role transition and adjustment, and 6) other specifics as defined by either party. Written evaluative comments are required at various times, depending on the educational program. Some programs require biweekly telephone conferences along with a written report brought by the learner to the program/learner biweekly conference. In this way, the learner and the preceptor know what is being discussed and program faculty are kept informed. There are no secrets in adult education—all evaluations need to be open and agreed upon by both the evaluator and the person being evaluated. This is the foundation for ongoing peer review of one's clinical practice, and must be modeled throughout the educational program. This openness in performance evaluation also eliminates the sometimes negative attacks on personality and style of either teacher or learner, and focuses the evaluation where it should be—on performance of expected outcomes.

A couple of precautionary notes are offered here for consideration by novice teachers. First of all, it is helpful for educational programs to clearly state that class/seminars take precedent over extended clinical time. This means that the learner cannot skip class because s/he was up all night with a birth, nor decide that s/he prefers to go the primary care site rather than attend class. This does not mean, however, that program faculty are unwilling to make an exception to this class time rule if clinical learning needs to take precedent. What helps in communication of such needs is when the learner and/or preceptor obtain prior approval from the course coordinator for missing class time to take advantage of needed clinical experience. Midwifery learners have a special need to learn early in their careers how to balance the 24/7 demands of the practice role with other aspects of their daily lives, including preparation for and attending class. Faculty can assist the learner in developing these skills by offering suggestions that have worked for others as well as themselves.

Primary care faculty often arrange for mid-semester and final site visits during which they do formative and summative evaluation of learner progress in collaboration with the clinical teachers. There are several formats for such visits, and offer time to discuss preceptor and site issues as well as learner progress. In this way, program faculty offer their wisdom and expertise (payment in kind) as well as a sympathetic ear as they also gain wisdom and expertise from practitioners in the clinical arena. A final written evaluation by the designated primary preceptor is prepared by the practice staff, shared with the learner, discussed, and signed by both preceptor and learner before it is sent to the university. Evaluative comments are then incorporated as appropriate into the graduate's end of program evaluation.

Stage IV: Evaluation

The final stage of utilization of clinical sites is evaluation. Evaluation takes several forms, including learner evaluation of the site as well as by the clinical teachers in that site. Evaluation forms can be helpful to direct the learner to comment on such things as adequacy of orientation to the site, physical facilities, communication effectiveness, availability of preceptors, and support of patients for learning. Verbal and/or written evaluation of the overall experience of having learners in the practice site is requested from the practice personnel, especially the primary preceptor. Comments on communication strategies used and their effectiveness, support of the program faculty for carrying out the clinical teaching role, and interest in continuing the clinical affiliation are encouraged. Suggestions for improving the program/clinical agency process are also encouraged, and plans should be made for the next placement of learners as appropriate.

Success in establishing and maintaining clinical sites for learning APN and midwifery practice is fostered by human contact, mutual agreement on goals and roles, and mutual respect of both program faculty and clinician roles based on shared understanding of what these roles demand of the individual. The preparation of APNs and midwives can only be accomplished with the collaborative partnership of academic and clinical personnel. It is the responsibility of the academic program to initiate and maintain this partnership.

AGENCY CONTRACTS AND NEGOTIATION

The need for a written contract is determined by the educational institution. If required, it is normal for the institution to insist on acceptance of its standard contract with minimal changes made. If the clinical site requires its own contract, the program director enters into a period of intense negotiation with lawyers representing both institutions. Knowing the sequence of signing these agreements (university first, then practice or vice versa) facilitates the process. Some health professional schools have a separate department for handling such negotiations, but they must be initiated and followed closely by program faculty as well. Given that learners will not be allowed in the clinical site without a signed agreement, this followup is essential to the well being of the program.

As noted earlier, the agency agreement or contract will include wording on indemnification of the clinical site and staff from errors made by learners. This agreement also makes reference to responsibilities of both parties (university and clinical site) in relation to placement of the university's learners in that setting, and includes a start and end date. The reader is encouraged to become very familiar with the academic unit's requirements for clinical agreements with sites/agencies and to take the needed steps to make sure these requirements are met.

In addition, it is vital to know approximately how long the contract process normally takes from initiation to completion so that this time can be factored into the assignments of learners to that site.

SELECTION CRITERIA FOR SITES AND PRECEPTORS

The criteria for selection of clinical sites and preceptors may vary. In general, an APN or midwifery program will select those clinical sites/practices that offer sufficient patient case mix and volume so that the learner can meet the expected competencies in clinical practice. Practices known for quality care and patient satisfaction are ideal, but not every site used for learning will meet this ideal on a daily basis. Here it is important to understand that the reality of clinical practice is what the learner needs, and to respect those clinicians who continue to do their best under very adverse conditions—whether caused by the setting, volume, or intensity of patient needs. As noted earlier, it is important for the academic program to consider whether the practice has a peer review process in place that is used on a regular basis, whether it is externally reviewed and accredited, and what the image of the practice is in the community where it is located. Proximity to the academic setting is important for some programs, while others use very distant sites for their learners.

Selection of clinical teachers or preceptors from the practice setting is based on several criteria. First of all, the preceptor must be licensed/legally able to practice. If a joint appointment is being considered, the preceptor must meet the academic requirements set by the university (usually a minimum of a master's degree). It is also important to check with accreditation agencies to determine whether they set additional criteria for those teaching in a clinical discipline. For example, a relatively new criteria for faculty and preceptors set by the Division of Accreditation of the American College of Nurse-Midwives (ACNM) requires that the nurse-midwife/midwife teacher "have preparation for teaching (include both didactic and clinical teaching)" (ACNM, 1998). In addition, the ACNM Division of Accreditation requires that all nurse-midwives/midwives be nationally certified by the ACNM Certification Corporation (ACC), have a minimum of a master's degree, have at least 1 year of clinical experience as a nurse-midwife/midwife prior to teaching, and demonstrate evidence of currency in practice. Other educational programs may require verification of licensure and will call the National Practitioner Data Bank to determine if the health professional (physician, nurse practitioner, or midwife) has a record of legal actions against them. Whatever the criteria, the teacher needs to know them and gather the needed data on each preceptor/clinical teacher.

PREPARATION OF PRECEPTORS

The preparation of clinicians as clinical teachers or preceptors is an important step in developing and implementing a successful APN or midwifery program (Hayes, 1994). Included in this preparation are many of the content areas covered in this book, beginning with how people learn and how teachers in any venue can facilitate learning. For some, use of Benner's (1984) framework of moving the learner from novice to advanced beginner provides the context for thinking about teaching strategies and design of clinical learning opportunities. For others, reading (or providing copies of) selected articles on the role of the clinical teacher can be helpful in thinking about the role and assessing one's strengths and areas to work on in carrying out that role. Formal preparation for the clinical teaching role may take the form of workshops, a semester class, or a post-master's certificate program in teaching in addition to the more traditional graduate preparation in adult (higher) education. Appendix G addresses suggested guidelines for the preparation of clinical teachers. Whatever the preparation, the foundation must be built on expert clinical practice and intimate knowledge of the educational program (curriculum, sequencing, performance outcomes), along with a clear definition of both teacher and learner expectations in the clinical setting.

The following is an overview of expectations of both teachers and learners in a clinical setting. It has been successfully used by the authors for several decades. It is a guide offered for novice teachers and new programs that can be modified to meet the current needs of a particular program. It is strongly recommended that such guidelines be constructed jointly with clinical and academic teachers, be written, and periodically reviewed and updated.

Education Program Expectations of Learners in Clinical Setting

The Learner functioning in a clinical setting will:

1. Be responsible for his/her own learning by:
    a. Preparing for each clinical assignment through reading, reviewing prior practice, and goals learning.
    b. Defining current learning needs clearly.
    c. Discussing learning needs with clinical teacher at beginning of each session.
    d. Seeking direction from clinical teacher in choosing appropriate clinical experiences to meet the day's learning goals.
    e. Sharing knowledge/experience deficits, if any, with clinical teacher at beginning of assigned clinical session.

    f. Evaluating own progress daily according to critical decision-making process and learning outcomes, and obtaining validation of self-evaluation from clinical teacher.

2. Demonstrate knowledge of and sensitivity to personnel and setting policies and procedures.
3. Know and practice within written nurse-midwifery/nurse practitioner policies and procedures.
4. Carry out assigned caregiving in a professional manner at all times.
5. Be responsible and accountable for learning and caregiving.
6. Notify proper authority in advance if s/he needs to be absent from clinical session for any reason.
7. Maintain and update clinical evaluation tool, have it available at all times, and maintain up-to-date statistics on clinical experiences as required by program.
8. Communicate progress to clinical teacher and course coordinator.
9. Evaluate clinical teacher's performance in teaching/evaluation, sharing evaluation with the clinical teacher, and obtaining his/her signature before bringing to course coordinator.
10. Evaluate specific effectiveness and characteristics of clinical site at end of rotation and turn in to course coordinator.

Education Program Expectations of Teachers in Clinical Setting

The teacher in a clinical setting will be:

1. Accepting of and committed to the philosophy of adult education espoused by the APN or midwifery educational program.
2. Accepting of the responsibilities of the clinical teacher including:
    a. Knowledge and support of the curriculum facilitated by:
        1. Having and reviewing copies of all course materials, seminar schedules, and updated bibliographies received from program.
        2. Knowledge of theoretical guidelines/timetables for expected learner progress.
        3. In-service/journal clubs at clinical faculty meetings.
    b. Knowledge and support of individual learner's needs and outcomes as defined by the learner and confirmed by course coordinator, facilitated by:
        1. Understanding how adults learn and types of learner behaviors.
        2. Flexibility and/or ability to change, based on learner needs.

      3. Site visits negotiated with program faculty.

      4. Identifying learning needs and deficits early and communicating these to the course or site coordinator in a timely manner.

      5. Awareness of individual learning styles when using learning plans and performance contracts.

      6. Telephone availability (established contact time, dates, etc.).

  c. Provision and delineation of the boundaries of safe practice in the setting and clear and repeated communication of these to the learner and program staff.

  d. Selection of appropriate clinical learning situations for level of learner in collaboration with course or site coordinator.

      1. Recognize need for special experiences for individual learners.

      2. Explore with learner his/her reasons for decline of a particular experience and handle appropriately.

  e. Support of learner's approach to APN or midwifery practice as long as it meets criteria of safety and minimal discomfort to the patient and is supported by valid rationale, given the realities of the setting.

  f. Provision of own theoretical rationale for clinical decisions and practice when requested or needed by the learner.

  g. Supervision of the learner's clinical practice and co-signing patient records after review.

  h. Evaluation of learner performance based on stated outcomes in pre- and post-conferences, completing evaluation tool according to program directions, and using criteria of safety, accuracy of findings, and minimal discomfort for the patient.

  i. Communication with course coordinator concerning progress of learning.

      1. Set times for telephone contact and report using suggested format.

      2. Attendance at clinical faculty meetings held at University.

      3. In sites where multiple clinicians participate in guidance and evaluation of learner progress, work together as group to evaluate progress before reporting to learner and program faculty.

3. Aware and accept that the role of clinical teacher requires one's undivided attention and that the clinical teacher may need to make alternate arrangements if expected to see a normal caseload simultaneously with teaching.

4. An active participant in evaluation of the APN or midwifery curriculum as facilitated by the academic setting.

5. Willing to be evaluated as a clinical teacher, review that evaluation, comment, and sign as evidence of review and discussion.

6. An active participant in activities that support an up-to-date-knowledge and practice base.

SUMMARY

The administrative details in establishing and maintaining a positive clinical learning environment for APN and midwifery learners are an important part of the role of any teacher. Successful preparation of the next generation of advanced practice nurses and midwives requires exposure to a variety of expert clinicians and patients in a variety of settings for care. When careful, deliberate attention is paid to the development and maintenance of clinical sites and clinical teachers, the reward will be graduation of competent, compassionate graduates.

REFLECTIONS

Think about your first exposure to a learner needing clinical guidance and help in knowing how to provide the care that you are expert in providing. What were your first thoughts about sharing patients with a new learner? What kind of support did your practice setting offer that made teaching others to do what you do possible and even fun?

What are the legal requirements for contracts in your academic or clinical setting? Who is responsible for making sure these are met? What is your role in establishing and maintaining clinical practice sites for your learners? How have you balanced the teaching and administrative details of your role with your love of practice?

REFERENCES

American College of Nurse-Midwives. (1998). *Criteria for accreditation of education programs in nurse-midwifery and midwifery.* Washington, DC: Author.

Beebe, J. E. (1980). Initiation and maintenance of clinical learning sites in nurse-midwifery. *Journal of Nurse-Midwifery, 25*(1), 29–32.

Benner, P. (1984). *From novice to expert: Excellence and power in clinical nursing practice.* Menlo Park, CA: Addison-Wesley.

Blanchard, K. (1985). *Situational leadership II.* Escondido, CA: Blanchard Training and Development Corporation.

Hayes, E. (1994). Helping preceptors mentor the next generation of nurse practitioners. *Nurse Practitioner, 19*(6), 62–66.

LeBlanc, R. (1999). Good teaching: The top ten requirements. *The Teaching Professor* (Sample Issue).

SELECTED BIBLIOGRAPHY

Atack, L., Comaco, M., Kenny, R., LaBelle, N., & Miller, D. (2000). Student and staff relationships in a clinical practice model: Impact on learning. *Journal of Nursing Education, 39*(9), 387–392.

Flager, S., Loper-Powers, S., & Spitzer, A. (1988). Clinical teaching is more than evaluation alone. *Journal of Nursing Education, 27*(8), 342–348.

Haukenes, E., & Hollahan, M. (1983). The selection of clinical learning experiences in the nursing curriculum. *Journal of Nursing Education, 22*(9), 351–356.

Oermann, M. H. (1998). Role strain of clinical nursing faculty. *Journal of Professional Nursing, 14*(6), 329–334.

Okafor, C. (1992). Criteria for the selection of experiences and content in midwifery education. *International Journal of Gynecology & Obstetrics, 38*(suppl.), S59–S62.

Reilly, D. E., & Oermann, M. H. (1992a). Preceptorship. In *Clinical teaching in nursing education* (pp. 196–200). New York: National League for Nursing.

Reilly, D. E., & Oermann, M. H. (1992b). *Clinical teaching in nursing education*. New York: National League for Nursing.

Tanner, C. A. (1994). On clinical teaching. *Journal of Nursing Education, 33*(9), 387–388.

CHAPTER 14

Academic Responsibilities of Teachers

It is a curious life we lead, the life of scholarship. Difficult and demanding, most certainly; frustrating, far too often for comfort; poorly rewarded in material terms; and calling for a great deal of spiritual stamina.

—G. Highet,
The Immortal Profession

SUGGESTED OUTCOMES FOR THIS CHAPTER

At the end of this chapter, the reader will be able to

1. describe the integrated roles and responsibilities of teacher, scholar, and clinician; and
2. define the levels/types of academic appointments, including the general criteria for appointment, promotion, and tenure in your university.

INTRODUCTION

When an individual makes the career decision to begin teaching formally within an academic program, whether advanced practice nursing or midwifery, it is a life changing event (Locasto, 1989; Peters, 1987). Hours of work, responsibilities, loyalties, and expectations change. Most of us made the decision to teach after some years of clinical practice. Some decided that the more controlled environment of teaching was preferable to the 24/7 practice of a clinician. Others made the decision after much thought and reflection on their commitment to the advancement of the profession through preparation of the next generation of clinicians. Teaching others to do what you do helps to ensure that many more health and illness care needs will be met than you alone could meet. Teaching others to do what you do also means that you have a say in the quality of advanced practice nursing and midwifery now and in the future. However, learning to teach and carrying out the academic responsibilities inherent in the university program may be quite new. This chapter will focus on what it means to teach in an academic setting, and briefly present some of the common academic expectations.

INTEGRATED ROLES AND RESPONSIBILITIES

Academia has many requirements and commitments in its search for truth and understanding. Academics, for the purposes of discussion in this chapter, are defined as those individuals who are employed by an institution of higher learning, whether it be a college or university, full or part time. An institution of higher learning or academic institution is commonly defined as a university or college accredited by an institutional accrediting agency recognized by the U.S. Department of Education (American College of Nurse Midwives [ACNM], 1999). Some examples of accrediting agencies include state or regional boards of education, the National League for Nursing (NLN), the Commission on Certification of Nursing Education (CCNE) or the American College of Nurse-Midwives Division of Accreditation (ACNM DOA).

In most health professions programs, academics are expected to meet a tripartite mission of education, research, and practice. As one will note in the next section, there are a variety of levels and types of academic appointments and each carries specific responsibilities. There are, however, common expectations of those who choose to teach in a clinical discipline. These expectations will be discussed in relation to the three missions of education, research, and practice.

Roles and Responsibilities of Teacher

The roles and responsibilities of teaching in advanced practice nursing and midwifery are similar to those in any of the health professions programs. Leafing through this book offers one perspective on the teaching role and responsibilities, including defining one's philosophy of adult education, the design, implementation and evaluation of curriculum, preparation of course materials, teaching and evaluation in the classroom and clinical settings, and establishing and maintaining clinical sites.

Other teacher responsibilities alluded to throughout the text include advisement of learners, mentoring others, and maintaining one's competence in theory as well as clinical practice. Marketing, recruitment, and admission of each class of learners is also a vital part of the role of the academic teacher, though often supported by university or college personnel with preparation in these areas. However, the advanced practice nurse or midwife teacher should never underestimate the importance of her/his presence in the recruitment and admission of applicants, as this affords the unique opportunity to demonstrate enthusiasm and describe the professional role in ways that non-nurse or midwife staff cannot do.

Preparation for the teaching role is important as reinforced throughout this text. Attitude toward and enthusiasm for teaching are also important. Nugent, Bradshaw, and Kito (1999) found that formal education courses and prior teaching experience led to greater levels of self-efficacy—the belief in one's ability to teach and to influence others to learn—in new nurse teachers (Ashton, 1984; Bandura, 1977; Guskey & Passaro, 1994). However, many teachers in advanced practice nursing or midwifery programs have not had the luxury of formal teaching preparation before being called upon or volunteering to teach—usually in the clinical area. Clinical teaching experience is an important base for academic teaching, and it has been discussed how workshops for preceptors can facilitate one's effectiveness as a clinical teacher. Many teachers have learned by doing and watching others and some have the benefit of mentors for their teaching development. All of these methods for learning and developing the teacher role are important (Daloz, 1986; Gelmon, 1999; Valiga & Streubert, 1991).

Roles and Responsibilities of Scholar

Academia requires a scholarly approach to teaching and practice from everyone who works in this setting (Sherman, Armistead, Fowler, Barksdale, & Reif, 1987). Scholarship can take several forms, including research, professional writing, and oral presentation of current trends and science at professional meetings. Research may be targeted to the basic sciences (bench scientist), to the design and testing of drugs or interventions in clinical practice, or to the use of large data sets to determine health and social policy effectiveness. The involvement of human subjects in research requires strict attention/adherence to the rules and regulations of protecting these individuals with, at minimum, free and informed consent for participation. Advanced practice nurses and midwives may begin their research development as the person who helps define and frame the clinical research question, or as one of the data collectors.

Publication of research findings is expected, and the new scholar often looks to a variety of senior researchers or works as a part of a research team as they learn how to design, carry out, and write about their clinical study. Scholarly writing can also come from direct clinical practice or related disciplines to the advanced practice nurse or midwife, such as health care ethics. The new academic often begins their scholarly writing based on the familiar aspects of clinical practice. The ability to read, synthesize, critique, and write about the scientific bases of nursing or midwifery practice is inherent in the scholarly expectations of the academic. Learning how to write for publication takes practice, practice, practice. It also requires one to have a good sense of self as it is rare that an article will be accepted for publication on the first try. In many of the research intensive universities, scholarly writing is a given and there are often senior faculty who will assist the novice teacher with their writing and scholarly development.

Presentations at professional meetings are a good way to begin one's trajectory of scholarship in nursing and midwifery. One of the author's mentors encouraged her to turn every presentation into an article for publication in recognition of the extensive reading, writing, and preparation that needs to precede any public presentation. This proved to be helpful in building a curriculum vita worthy of appointment and promotion in several universities. Oral or poster presentations also provide excellent experience in presenting new and often complex information in a way that can be easily understood—a very important skill for the teacher in both classroom and clinical settings. Presenting on clinical topics at professional meetings also serves to keep the teacher/clinician up to date in their area of specialization, another essential attribute of a good teacher. Whatever type of scholarly activity one chooses, it should be focused on an area of interest that will develop over time. This interest provides the sustaining motivation to continue to develop one's skills and expertise in scholarly productivity.

Roles and Responsibilities of Clinician

When one is teaching in a clinical discipline, it is vital to maintain both competence and confidence in that area of practice. Learners will challenge every teacher's competence as they seek out a clinician they can trust while they are learning to become both competent and confident. Much learning time is wasted when academics have lost touch with the current world of practice in their discipline, as the learner will immediately know this and begin to challenge every word. This means the learner is spending more time on checking whether the teacher really knows anything and less time on learning how to be a good clinician. A novice learner also needs a competent teacher/clinician as modeling is often the first way of defining the role and responsibilities of an advanced practice nurse or midwife.

When one takes on the full academic role and responsibilities in a practice discipline, it is vital to decide how much clinical practice with and without students is needed to maintain one's competence. If the academic program carries responsibility for maintaining a caseload of patients, it is usually expected that all teachers participate in that practice. If the academic program uses all affiliated agencies for clinical placement of learners, it may be possible to assign oneself a day a week to one of these settings to maintain one's skills or to keep up with the progress of learning among one's students. A general rule of thumb that has worked for the authors is to make sure that one is competent in practice in the area of academic teaching; for example, if one is responsible for the antepartum course in a given semester, their practice commitment would ideally be carried out in an antepartum setting. Some new teachers wish to maintain a significant clinical practice while teaching in the classroom as they love and feel most confident in working with patients. Expert teachers often carry a minimum of clinical practice, primarily because as they move along the academic pathway, increasing expectations for scholarship and university service take up more time.

Whatever the academic institution you are working in, there is a professional as well as institutional expectation that the tripartite mission of education, scholarship, and practice will be an integral part of your daily life. The authors have found it helpful to look beyond a single day or week or month when achieving such a mission. In other words, novice teachers often benefit from an emphasis on learning the educator role first while maintaining the practice role. As the teacher matures, more and more scholarship is expected and natural based on one's ever-expanding expertise in the discipline. Expert teachers who are also expert clinicians may design their academic appointment with a focus on research and scholarly writing without fear of losing either their expertise in teaching or practice. All three roles are important to the future of advanced practice nursing and midwifery, and each will receive a variable level of attention depending on the nature of the academic institution and the type of academic appointment.

LEVEL/TYPES OF ACADEMIC APPOINTMENTS

The levels and types of academic appointments will vary from university to university, and sometimes, within the schools of one university or college. As when seeking any change of employment, the individual is urged to have a frank discussion during interview regarding the levels and types of academic appointments available to them, given their credentials. It is important to know the length of the yearly appointment (9, 10, 11, or 12 months), length of initial contract (1–3 years), criteria for reappointment, and whether tenure is a possible option now or in the future, in addition to understanding expectations for carrying out the position. Several types of appointments are discussed below.

Appointments for Master's Prepared Teachers

Master's prepared teachers who are expert clinicians form the backbone of teaching in advanced practice nursing and midwifery, especially in those programs that result in a master's degree upon completion. Academic institutions offering certificate programs in midwifery or advanced practice nursing also require the master's degree as a minimum credential for the teacher, both from an educational point of view and to meet external accrediting agency requirements (ACNM, 1999). While there is a place for an expert clinician without a graduate degree, usually as clinical preceptor, they would rarely be given an academic appointment.

In some universities, master's prepared nursing or midwifery teachers are given an appointment as a lecturer (titles will vary from one institution to another) as distinct from the more commonly used assistant, associate, or full professor ranks accorded only to those with an earned doctorate. Many academic institutions, however, do use the professorial ranks with master's prepared individuals while others will attach the prefix of "clinical" to each to distinguish the clinical assistant professor (master's prepared) from the assistant professor (doctorally prepared). Institutions with a strong educational mission and less emphasis on research in nursing are those that tend to offer the professorial ranks to master's prepared individuals.

Depending on the size of the academic institution, its research classification, the number of other schools or departments included besides nursing, and the rules of procedure for appointment, promotion, and tenure, there can be a fair degree of creativity used in designing academic appointments for the master's prepared teacher. These will need the scrutiny of the human resources personnel along with agreement among faculty. One example comes from the academic home of the authors. Since the university limit for full time lecturers (master's prepared) was 3 years, the master's prepared teachers had to leave the university after this time and there was great turnover in program faculty in the APN and midwifery programs. A new appointment was created with a 7-year time limit to be used with full time master's prepared teacher-clinicians. The title was "Lecturer/ Clinical Specialist" and was designed especially for the nurse-midwifery and primary care nurse practitioner programs. This appointment category has afforded stability in those programs from both a curricular and teaching standpoint. In fact, several of the master's prepared clinician-teachers remained with the midwifery program for over 12 years by converting to part time status after 7 years. (Part time statuses in most academic institutions are annual appointments and can be repeated without limit provided the person contributes to the program and there are sufficient resources to support them.)

Appointments for Doctorally Prepared Teachers

An earned doctorate (ScD, DNSc, EdD, PhD) usually qualifies the holder for a professorial appointment within an academic institution. A first appointment to the academic ranks begins as an assistant professor. The assistant professor criteria and length of service without promotion vary from university to university. Criteria for reappointment and/or promotion tend to focus on teaching excellence and scholarly productivity at this level, with lesser emphasis on university, community, or professional service. In general, an initial appointment as an assistant professor will be for a 3- or 4-year term, with review for reappointment during the penulti-mate year. The total number of years one can stay in the assistant professor rank is normally 7 years, with promotion to associate professor by that time. Some universities will promote an assistant professor to the rank of associate professor without tenure, while others offer tenure with the associate or full professor level. Tenure award means that the university guarantees employment for the rest of one's career in that institution provided there remains a school or college and the faculty member performs within the stated norms of academia.

Appointment and/or promotion to associate professor or full professor is usually dependent on the extent of scholarly productivity and national/international reputa-tion in the discipline. Teaching excellence and service are still important, but often overshadowed by research and scholarship, especially in research intensive universities. Once a teacher moves to doctoral preparation and senior ranks, their direct teaching time is often limited by the other academic demands on their time. Likewise, practice time is very limited or nonexistent. Some advanced practice specialty areas in nursing still have a paucity of doctorally prepared teachers, hence the earlier statement that master's prepared teacher-clinicians are the backbone of this type of graduate education. This is true also in midwifery education, though the percentage of doctorally prepared midwives is much higher than the nursing average. Many are in clinical research, however, and thus not available to carry out the day-to-day teaching responsibilities.

For those individuals who wish to maintain their clinical excellence and also work in academic environments, universities have created an alternative to the tenure track professorial ranks. At the University of Pennsylvania School of Nursing, the name of this rank is "Clinician Educator" and it is reserved for those doctorally prepared individuals in the health schools (medicine, nursing, dentistry) who share their academic appointment with a practice agency. They are full time employees of the University with part of their salary reimbursed by the clinical agency.

Appointments for Clinicians/Preceptors

Individuals who work in a practice setting as clinicians and agree to take advanced practice nursing and midwifery learners from a university program, often without salary remuneration, can be offered an official appointment at most universities. The titles and credentials for such appointments do vary, with the most common title being either clinical instructor or preceptor. The most common requirement is a minimum of a master's degree (usually must be in nursing if the program resides within a college or school of nursing). These university appointments are often seen as a valuable reward that recognizes the importance of this clinician's role in preparing new practitioners. For those expert clinicians who do not meet the academic unit's criteria for appointment, a nicely worded and framed certificate of appreciation has been used with success and appreciation. The expectations of clinical instructors and/or preceptors must be clearly defined and agreed upon by both the academic faculty and clinician (see chapter 13 for detailed discussion of program expectations of teachers in a clinical setting).

SUMMARY

There are several commonalities within the discussion of academic appointments and expectations that can be helpful for the new teacher. First of all, know the criteria for appointment, reappointment, and promotion for each type of appointment in your academic setting. Secondly, determine who the person is who has final say over hiring new teachers, evaluating their performance, and determining who will continue and what they will be paid. Conditions of appointment are important for everyone, and knowing these before recruiting expert clinicians is vital. Thirdly, prepare, practice, evaluate, and prepare some more, for effective teaching and scholarship come with doing, just as effective advanced practice nursing and midwifery come with doing.

Another aspect of academic responsibilities relates to the need for balance between the various potentially conflicting loyalties of the teacher. These loyalties begin with learning the teaching role and move quickly to responsibility to the learners, the clinical settings, the profession, as well as to the academic setting, with its need to pursue and extend the boundaries of both the science and art of the practice of nursing and midwifery. A new teacher in an academic setting may have selected this career pathway after a clinical role, so loyalty to one's patients in the past and present may cause conflict or lack of balance in one's personal as well as professional life. Whatever the loyalty, the new teacher needs to set realistic goals for self, including realistic learning time, preparation time, and scholarly time, in collaboration with a senior academic/program coordinator who agrees with these goals and time frame.

Finally, search for a mentor (or several) early in your career. As noted by Daloz (1986), mentoring involves three distinct roles or responsibilities—those of supporter, challenger, and visionary. A supporter affirms your teaching skills and performance, and assists you to set realistic goals and change needed teacher behaviors. A challenger is needed to push you outside your comfort zone and experiment with new ways of teaching and new approaches to scholarship. A visionary works with you to illumine long range goals and to sketch your career dreams that are followed with strategic steps in accomplishing those dreams (McCloskey & Grace, 1990). It is the responsibility of senior academics to mentor junior faculty, and this is especially needed in advanced practice nursing and midwifery educational programs so that knowledgeable, expert clinicians become knowledgeable, expert teachers, scholars, and university citizens.

REFLECTIONS

Think about your first introduction to academic faculty and the university you attended for your own advanced practice nursing of midwifery preparation. Reflect on the various ways your teachers were able to balance multiple demands on their time and still be present for the learners. What are some of the strategies you will or have used to adjust to the many demands of being an academic? Who are your mentors for teaching, scholarship, and professional service? What do you especially like about being an academic? What career development strategies have you used to define your near and long-term future in advanced practice or midwifery, and what place does academic teaching have in that plan?

REFERENCES

American College of Nurse-Midwives. (1999). *ACNM Division of Accreditation policies and procedures manual.* Washington, DC: Author. Available on-line: http://www. ACNM.org/educ/

Ashton, P. (1984). Teacher efficacy: A motivational paradigm for effective teacher education. *Journal of Teacher Education, 35*(5), 28–32.

Bandura, A. (1977). Self-efficacy: Toward a unifying theory of behavior change. *Psychological Review, 84,* 191–215.

Daloz, L. (1986). *Effective teaching and mentoring.* Menlo Park, CA: Jossey-Bass.

Gelmon, S. B. (1999). Promoting teaching competency and effectiveness for the 21st century. *American Association of Nurse Anesthetists Journal, 67*(5), 409–416.

Guskey, T. R., & Passaro, P. D. (1994). Teacher efficacy: A study of construct dimensions. *American Educational Research Journal, 31,* 627–643.

Highet, G. (1976). *The immortal profession.* New York: Weybright and Talley.

Locasto, L. W. (1989). Reality shock in the nurse-educator. *Journal of Nursing Education, 28*(2), 79–81.

McCloskey, J. C., & Grace, H. K. (1990). *Current issues in nursing* (3rd ed.). St. Louis: Mosby.

Nugent, K. E., Bradshaw, M. J., & Kito, N. (1999). Teacher self-efficacy in new nurse educators. *Journal of Professional Nursing, 15*(4), 229–237.

Peters, T. (1987). *Thriving on chaos*. New York: Harper & Row.
Sherman, T. M., Armistead, L. P., Fowler, F., Barksdale, M. A., & Reif, G. (1987). The quest for excellence in university teaching. *Journal of Higher Education, 48*, 66–84.
Valiga, T., & Streubert, H. J. (1991). *Nurse educator in academia: Strategies for success*. New York: Springer Publishing.

CHAPTER 15

Promoting Academic Integrity

Michele A. Goldfarb, Esq.

SUGGESTED OUTCOMES FOR THIS CHAPTER

At the end of this chapter, the reader will be able to

1. discuss codes of academic integrity and how they affect the learner and teacher in a university setting, and
2. identify potential situations with learners and teachers that can raise legal concerns.

INTRODUCTION

Whether in the individual classroom, laboratory, or clinic, in institutions of higher education as a whole, or in society in general, the prospect that large numbers of students are engaging in multiple acts of academic dishonesty casts a long and troubling shadow. The prevalence of academic dishonesty is alarming to many who fear that our schools are fashioning scholars and professionals of questionable worth. Worse still, perhaps, is the disturbing notion that American colleges and universities are failing in their responsibility to produce principled citizens of the nation and, ultimately, the globe. If we can extrapolate to the larger culture from what we know about levels of academic dishonesty among college students, if college is the dry run for our young people, then it is critical that institutions of higher learning promote ethical values and respond to breaches of established standards of conduct in an effective, thoughtful manner.

This chapter is intended to provide guidance on how best to promote academic integrity and minimize opportunities for academic dishonesty. Further, it offers general advice on legal principles and sound institutional practice in order to help faculty exercise good judgment in those realms. The guidelines here are not, however, a substitute for competent legal counsel for specific situations.

EXTENT OF THE PROBLEM

Research has been conducted on a national scale over the past several decades attempting to identify levels of cheating among college students (McCabe & Trevino, 1993). The surveys undertaken involved thousands of students at dozens of selective institutions of higher education. The results of this research indicate a widespread problem. More than 75% of students admit to cheating one or more times in their college careers. About 25% self-report more than three incidents of cheating during college (Kibler, 1995). Perhaps one of the most disconcerting results in the research indicates that over 80% of those surveyed profess to thinking that under no circumstances is cheating justified (McCabe, 1993).

Moreover, as one might hypothesize, this behavior may not have originated in college. A survey of "High Achievers" conducted by Who's Who Among High School Students during 1992–1993 indicated that nearly 80% self-reported some form of dishonesty, and almost half had cheated on an exam or quiz (Kibler, 1995).

What is the meaning of all this? Why do students cheat? Where does it come from? What motivates them? What follows is some speculation about the roots of the problem.

INFLUENCES ON ACADEMIC INTEGRITY

Numerous factors influence the occurrence of academic dishonesty and may account for what appears to be unacceptably poor adherence to principles of honesty and integrity in scholarship and other academic work. Some of these influences are general, almost global, in nature. Others are institutional, and still more involve group and personal perceptions and realities. However, if we are to effectively address the issue of academic dishonesty, some discussion and appreciation of its underlying causes must occur.

Some attribute the seeming rise in academic dishonesty to shifts in values occurring across our entire social, cultural, and political environment (Gehring, Nuss, & Pavela, 1986). These societal shifts place greater (arguably undue) emphasis on successful competition, elevate individual concerns over community ones, and measure achievement in material wealth and other concrete indicia. Some blame current levels of academic dishonesty on our apparently high regard for "winning" at any cost. In the realm of academic integrity this translates into a feeling that crafty cheating is gutsy and almost admirable and, at any rate, amusing (Dunn, 1999).

Competition, with its external realities and internal consequences, is often cited as a major contributor to academic dishonesty. There is increased competition for admission into selective graduate programs and professional schools (Gehring et al., 1986). Students face heightened competition and expectations in the college admissions process at an earlier age (Gardner, 1996). Along with this competition comes pressure from families for students to "make good" on an educational investment and internal pressure for students to "have something to show" for sacrifices families have made along the way.

Some speculate that the excessive significance placed on scores, grades, and other somewhat standardized measures of accomplishment makes cheating almost inevitable since the underlying message communicated serves to devalue the learning process and reward only quantifiable outcomes (Shapiro, 2000).

On an institutional level, academic dishonesty is attributed to several more specific factors. Students complain that expectations and standards are poorly defined and badly communicated and that it is often not clear what constitutes dishonest behavior. In addition, students feel disengaged from the educational process in several ways. To many the content of the curriculum feels disconnected from perceived career needs (Gehring et al., 1986). Large classes taught by less experienced, less esteemed instructors can be demoralizing and can lead students to distance themselves from their coursework and more easily rationalize dishonesty. Related to this is the perception that the issue of academic integrity lacks importance to faculty, either because faculty rarely mention it or seem to ignore it when it occurs. Such perceptions appear to negatively influence levels of integrity at surveyed institutions (Kibler, 1995).

Along similar lines, and important for developing constructive institutional responses other factors have been identified as having an adverse impact on academic honesty. A decrease in the levels of cheating is more likely when students perceive that the institution/faculty take integrity seriously, that detection is probable, and that serious negative consequences will be imposed if cheating is detected (McCabe & Trevino, 1996). In other words, if risks are perceived as minimal, the other pressures at play make it more likely that our students will succumb to academic dishonesty.

FACULTY REACTIONS TO THE ACADEMIC INTEGRITY ISSUE

Everyone affiliated with higher education, particularly in the area of student affairs and discipline, knows that, relatively speaking, very few cases of academic dishonesty are handled through formal institutional channels. Many faculty have never reported a case of academic dishonesty and many express a frank reluctance to do so (Schneider, 1999). Faculty reactions to the academic integrity issue cover a broad spectrum. Many resist the issue in their classrooms and syllabi for fear of appearing mistrustful and negative. Faculty often state that highlighting the possibility of academic dishonesty alters their relationship with their students, turning them more into monitors or watchdogs than scholars and educators. Some frankly don't want to be bothered, perceiving (sometimes quite accurately) campus disciplinary systems to be burdensome and time consuming.

Furthermore, with respect to campus disciplinary responses, faculty impressions run the gamut. Many feel that university-imposed sanctions are too lenient and diminish the seriousness of the infraction. On the other hand, many others think that their university is overly punitive and are loathe to be involved in an accusation and process that might have lasting, even lifelong, consequences for the student. Finally, some faculty perceive a lack of support in their college administrations and worry that pressure from outside influences can cause the administration to unfairly side with the student.

What feedback can we give to faculty with respect to their overall hesitation to respond to incidents of academic dishonesty? Part of the answer lies in the data referred to in the previous section, i.e., that levels of cheating are related to a perceived lack of institution interest and response. The greater the perceived risk of detection and consequences, the lower the likelihood of academic dishonesty (Kibler, 1995).

Moreover, institutional action is the only reliable method of tracking a student's behavior across the curriculum. A student whose dishonest behavior is undetected in one course, or subject to informal action (a faculty warning or an adjusted grade) in another, may be performing similarly in most of his courses, thus undermining the legitimacy of his or her entire educational record.

In addition, it is important to recognize the educational potential of requiring a student to answer for his or her unethical behavior. At the risk of sounding utopian, the institution is in the business of training future professionals and citizens and at least a component of that responsibility is to build a foundation for ethical decision-making. Every discipline has standards of intellectual honesty and professional ethics with which competent practitioners must comply. A student whose academic dishonesty has gone unaddressed or has been inadequately handled is at great risk for meeting professional standards in the future where the stakes may be much higher.

Finally, to the extent that faculty choose to handle academic integrity matters by their own unofficial rules, they run the risk of losing institutional protection (Kibler, Nuss, Paterson, & Pavela, 1988). In fact, the safest way to obtain successful protection from liability as a faculty member in an academic integrity matter is to know and follow institutional procedures in good faith.

GENERAL PRINCIPLES TO GUIDE FACULTY RESPONSE TO ACADEMIC DISHONESTY

A good starting point at any institution, whether public or private, is knowledge of institutional policies, procedures, and regulations. These policies are contained in handbooks addressed to faculty only as well as institution-wide publications. Two of the principal reasons for familiarity and compliance with these published rules are: 1) many of them reflect and embody applicable law, and 2) they can be and have been interpreted as an implied contract with students and failure to follow those rules involves a breach of contract (Mancla v. Brown University, 1998). Institutional policies and regulations are rules that the university has committed itself to honoring. Therefore, failure to follow articulated institution guidelines in good faith can be more problematic for a faculty member even if the motivation is the benign one of reaching more informal resolutions.

Another basic piece of important information is whether or not your institution is an "honor code school." Features that characterize honor code schools are honor pledges, unproctored examinations, student run honor boards/disciplinary systems, requirement to report violations and, often, automatic repercussions for even first-time violations. Not every feature occurs in every school with an honor code. In order to conform with the expectations and culture of your institution, you must understand the extent to which the institution has and enforces zero tolerance and reporting rules.

Other important institutional policies that faculty must be familiar with, and that are in place in most schools are policies regulating use of alcohol on campus, use of permissible conduct in university facilities (including classrooms), and use of the university name and equipment. Again, awareness of institutional expectations is fundamental.

Finally, faculty have particular affirmative responsibility in the area of making accommodations for students with physical and mental disabilities. At times, there will be lengthy, detailed departmental/institutional guidelines of accommodations that must be made for students with identified disabilities. Understanding your responsibilities in this domain goes far beyond the scope of this chapter. However, it is key for faculty and institutions to learn the scope and applicability of the Americans with Disabilities Act, by consulting with the Office of Civil Rights of the Department of Education and appropriate legal counsel.

Additional general principles involve issues about the confidentiality of student records and other privacy considerations. Both the Registrar's office and University Counsel are well informed regarding the management of student records and ordinarily inform faculty and other university officials about school policy and the requirements of law. As a general matter, student educational records should not be shared with anyone but the student except for certain limited exceptions (FERPA, 1999). In the realm of academic integrity in particular this general requirement plays out in certain specific ways. For example, posting of grades that can be personally linked to particular students (via names, social security numbers, or other identification indicia) is prohibited.

Furthermore, student disciplinary records in matters of academic integrity are protected. In such matters, common decency, requirements of law, and the need to preserve the integrity of the investigation dictate that the following precautions should be observed:

- Students should be informed privately if a matter of academic dishonesty is under investigation.
- All witnesses should be informed that the matter is confidential.
- Documents should be maintained in a secure location.
- Consult only school officials who have a legitimate educational interest in the matter.
- Discuss the matter only with those school officials charged with investigating and resolving the matter (along with appropriate department chairs, deans, or colleagues with a legitimate educational interest).

Faculty who follow the simple dictates of sound judgment, discretion, and appropriate consultation should be protected against allegations of improper disclosure and defamation (Kibler et al., 1988).

Before discussing the specific recommendations regarding ways to promote academic honesty, one final general guideline should be emphasized. Faculty expectations about course requirements, assignments, behavior in class, labs, and clinics should be clearly and specifically expressed. This will be discussed in greater detail below but clarity of requirements deserves stressing as an overarching principle for faculty.

Heightening Awareness/Educating Students

The following several sections of this chapter are designed to furnish suggestions for ways to increase awareness about academic integrity and to educate your students about your expectations and standards regarding ethical conduct in academic work. These suggestions are meant as helpful ideas and are not intended as formulas or requirements. Some suggestions are quite specific to the discipline or assignment, and some are common sense. They provide examples of ways to minimize temptation and opportunity for cheating and to impress upon students your commitment to their learning and self-discovery. The goal is to provide a variety of choices that can be adapted as appropriate to your course or discipline.

Suggestions:

- Address academic integrity in the syllabus, in the classroom, in the lab, during supervision sessions in the clinic. Place special emphasis on the subject during introductory classes, and just before examinations, papers, journals, etc., are due.

- Emphasize and answer questions about requirements and standards of conduct, particularly with respect to completion of research, homework assignments, and examinations.
- Provide specific negative examples of ways in which students have transgressed in the past in handling assignments for a particular course.
- Clarify the degree to which collaboration is permissible—both for group work and individual work. Provide a procedure should a dispute arise regarding group projects so that it can be resolved before accusations and further difficulties occur.
- Clarify whether it is permissible to use past examination questions, past examination answers, or lab reports, case studies, etc., prepared in previous years.
- Specify whether papers must be entirely new work or whether duplications/alterations/expansions of previous work are acceptable. State whether prior permission is required when a student intends to submit for credit a paper previously (or simultaneously) used to fulfill another course's requirement.
- Educate students about plagiarism where appropriate. Direct them to resources that provide definitions and examples. Explain the relevance of proper attribution and the importance of honestly integrating another's work into one's own thinking. Alert students that you are savvy about plagiarism and other abuses from electronic resources.
- Explain to students that violations of academic integrity standards will be confronted if detected and referred for investigation to the appropriate university office.
- Particularize the importance and relevance of integrity and ethics to your discipline, wherever possible.

Informing Yourself and Students About Academic Resources

Often a student who has transgressed in the realm of academic integrity is struggling with academic difficulties. Most campuses have a myriad of resources with which you should become familiar and to which students can be directed. These include academic support programs, tutoring and mentoring resources, computing and library help, and writing resource centers.

In addition, there are numerous excellent Internet resources on plagiarism. A quick search will reveal a number of these. Examples of excellent sites (at the time of this writing) are:

1. *http://www.northwestern.edu/uacc/plagiar.html*
2. *http://sja.ucdavis.edu/SJA/plagiarism.html#how*
3. *http://Alexia.lis.uiuc.edu/~janicke/plagiary.htm*

While these sites provide useful tools for the student struggling to "do it right," the real challenge, again, is to persuade students of the profound value to themselves and to you of participating in their education in an honest way.

Guidelines for Preventing or Minimizing Cheating

What follow are numerous practical recommendations of concrete things that can be done to reduce opportunities for academic dishonesty. Again, these suggestions are not formulaic nor are they necessarily innovative or crafty. Many appear in whole or in part on campus and faculty websites around the world. They are intended to catalog at a glance a group of strategies from which to choose those most applicable to your teaching needs.

Examinations

- Provide explicit instructions regarding what materials, aids, etc., can be used (e.g., programmable calculators, electronic organizers, cellular phones).
- Make use of reasonable seating arrangements and rooms of appropriate size.
- Consider refusing to give credit on correct answers unless all work is shown.
- Choose and train proctors carefully; have adequate number of proctors.
- Consider asking students to sign bluebooks attesting to compliance with academic integrity rules.
- Photocopy graded examinations before returning them to students. Alternatively photocopy a random sample of graded examinations and tell students you will be doing so; develop a required statement for students to sign attesting that they have not altered examinations submitted for regrades.
- Set up a process to handle late requests to take an examination at an alternate time so that you are not taken unaware by these requests. For example, decide how to handle illness on the morning of the examination or how to handle the claim that extracurricular activities interfered with time to study, leading to a late request to take an examination at another time.

Papers and Other Projects

Before listing the following suggestions, it is important to acknowledge that many of these recommendations entail additional work for faculty.

- Change and create new paper topics regularly; choose to assign narrow, specific subject matter, which diminishes the likelihood that generic papers on the topic are available in paper "warehouses," on the Internet, or elsewhere. The more unique and personal the assignments, the less likely is plagiarism.

- Photocopy good papers and keep a file of them (let colleagues know you have them).
- Require and review drafts, outlines, and research notes.
- Familiarize yourself with Internet "term paper mills"; know how to search them.
- Familiarize yourself with websites and computerized software designed to aid in the detection of plagiarism; learn how to operate the search tools necessary to detect plagiarism. There are several on-line articles with quick, explicit, and comprehensive instructions. These include the following:

    1. *http://www.vanguard.edu/rharris/antiplag.htm*
    2. *http://www.siu.edu/~cesl/teachers/uwfp.html*
    3. *http://newark.rutgers.edu/~ehrlich/plagiarism598.html*

Guidelines to Follow if You Witness Cheating in Progress

In order to properly confront what you believe to be cheating during the course of an in-progress examination, a few simple precepts prevail. These suggestions are intended to serve the following goals: interrupt the cheating, respectfully and discreetly confront the student(s) involved, reiterate your expectations to the rest of the class, preserve and memorialize any documentation of the event, and interfere as little as possible with the evaluation of the student's academic work until further investigation into the alleged misconduct can occur.

It is recommended that you:

- Remove any notes or other items a student is using impermissibly. Do so immediately. Save anything you confiscate. Make a note of what you have seen and what has been done.
- Instruct students to move apart, change seats, etc.
- Reiterate your examination-taking expectations, rules, and potential consequences.
- Permit the student(s) to complete an examination, even if you suspect cheating. Interrupt the suspected impermissible conduct, identify the student(s) involved, set their examinations aside at the end of the examination, record names, and keep a seating chart in order to identify and contact witnesses at a later time, if necessary.

What to Do After the Fact if You Suspect Academic Dishonesty

Some of the most difficult decisions that must be faced occur after an act of academic dishonesty is detected. It is extremely important that a faculty member proceed cautiously, judiciously, and with a heightened sensitivity to institutional rules and student privacy.

The first question that may come to mind, particularly with respect to written work, is how to know whether a paper submitted by a student is authentic. Several clues may signal a paper that has been plagiarized in whole or in part:

- The writing style, either sentence-to-sentence, or paragraph-to-paragraph, fluctuates inexplicably.
- The paper looks "too professional."
- The paper differs significantly from previous work submitted by the student, particularly from assignments written in class.
- The work is more sophisticated or accomplished than you would expect from the student.
- The paper, or parts of it, sound familiar. It may duplicate excellent work submitted in a previous semester or may be copied from authoritative texts with which you are familiar.
- Paper is written on a topic that is slightly (or entirely) off the subject matter of the course or of the assignment.

If your suspicions have been aroused in any of the preceding ways or if other dishonest conduct comes to your attention, the following course of action is recommended.

Consult

Unless you have had considerable experience in this arena before, you should try to consult with others at the institution about the appropriate next steps. When doing so, it is critical to keep in mind a student's privacy. In fact, most initial consultations can be done without mentioning a student's name at all, but by simply describing the situation. Likely sources of advice in this area include appropriate colleagues, department chairs, disciplinary officers, and, of course, policy and procedures manuals.

Address

Inform the student promptly and in private about the nature of your concerns. Even if you are convinced that a student has cheated or lied, treat him/her respectfully, professionally, and candidly. Approaching a student in this way diminishes the possibility that the matter will deteriorate into hostility and defensiveness. Experience indicates that a student approached straightforwardly is more likely to accept responsibility.

Always keep the original of any suspected work of academic dishonesty and return a copy to the student. If permitted and encouraged by your institution's procedural rules, meet with the student and let him/her know your specific concerns. Consider asking the student an open-ended question, such as "What do you have to say about this?" or "What is your response?"

If appropriate, try to determine how justified your concerns are. You may want to check a student's familiarity with the concepts, vocabulary, or references used in the suspicious paper. Consider asking about sources or requesting to see sources, research notes, outlines, previous drafts, etc.

Decide What to Do Next

Keep an open mind. You may learn enough from a student to reasonably conclude that your original suspicions are unsubstantiated. Furthermore, you should consider whether the problem is poor academic work or academic dishonesty. Consider academic support resources for a student who is struggling to act in accordance with the rules and needs help. Again, and most importantly, know and follow your institution's procedures. Finally, let the student know what you intend to do and what to expect next.

Grades

Each institution will have its own protocol with respect to how accusations and findings of academic dishonesty impact the assigning of a grade. Some schools keep the two processes entirely separate; others permit grades to be assigned as responses to violations of academic integrity. It is important not to assume that the two functions are either linked or entirely disconnected. Know what your institution permits or mandates in this regard.

CONCLUSION

Academic integrity is at the heart of every educational enterprise. Moreover, academic integrity does not mean merely the absence of crib sheets at examinations, adequate attribution in research papers, or authentic data in the lab. It is a commitment, from both faculty and students, to engage in ethical thinking, scholarship, and dialogue throughout the entire curriculum. One of the most hopeful signs that the academic community is meeting the challenge of unethical behavior is the move in many places to integrate ethical discourse in every discipline, every course. The expectation that this kind of discourse is as appropriate in an art history course as it is in an accounting course is spreading. The role of the faculty is not to supply answers, engage in self-righteous preaching or signal dire warnings of doom. Instead, faculty can guide discussions in which they, along with students, identify issues of ethical concern, grapple with the often diverse approaches to resolving those concerns, and together construct a framework from which ethical choices can be made. If students experience this as the understood norm by which faculty operate, they are far more likely to adapt their behavior and thinking to this norm. Infusing the campus community with this quality of ethical inquiry and mutually respectful behavior will ultimately be more effectual in furthering a goal of academic integrity than all other prevention and detection strategies combined.

REFLECTIONS

Think about the importance of integrity to the competent and successful performance of your profession. Reflect upon ways to convey how important integrity is to you, either in terms of academic integrity or in broader terms of the meaningful practice of advanced practice nursing and midwifery.

REFERENCES

Dunn, A. (1999, February 7). Welcome to the evil house of cheat. *Los Angeles Times Magazine*, p. 30. (Special millennium issue/education: The new moral morality).
FERPA. (1999). *Family Educational Rights and Privacy Act* (20 U.S.C. 1232g, 34 CFR 99).
Gardner, R., Jr. (1996, March 18). Give me Harvard or give me death. *New York Magazine*, p. 33.
Gehring, D., Nuss, E. M., & Pavela, G. (1986). *Issues and perspectives on academic integrity*. Columbus, OH: NAPSA, Inc.
Kibler, W. L. (1995, February). *Addressing student academic dishonesty and promoting academic integrity*. Paper presented at the 16th Annual Law and Higher Education Conference, Ashville, NC.
Kibler, W. L., Nuss, E. M., Paterson, B. G., & Pavela, G. (1988). *Academic integrity and student development: Legal issues/policy perspectives*. Ashville, NC: College Administration Publications, Inc.
Mancla v. Brown University, 135 F.3d 80 (1st Cir. 1998).
McCabe, D. L. (1993). Faculty responses to academic dishonesty: The influence of student honor codes. *Research in Higher Education, 34*(5), 647–658.
McCabe, D. L., & Trevino, L. K. (1993). Academic dishonesty: Honor codes and other contextual influences. *Journal of Higher Education, 64*(5), 522–538.
McCabe, D. L., & Trevino, L. K. (1996, January/February). What we know about cheating in college: Longitudinal trends and recent developments. *Change*, pp. 29–33.
Schneider, A. (1999). Why professors don't do more to stop students who cheat. *Chronicle of Higher Education*. Colloquy (http://www.chronicle.com/colloquy/aa/cheat/background.htm.)
Sharpiro, S. (2000, Sept./Oct.). Who is cheating whom? *Tikkun* (magazine). Vol. 15, No. 5, p. 21.

Appendix A

SCHEMA OF CURRICULUM DEVELOPMENT AND DESIGN

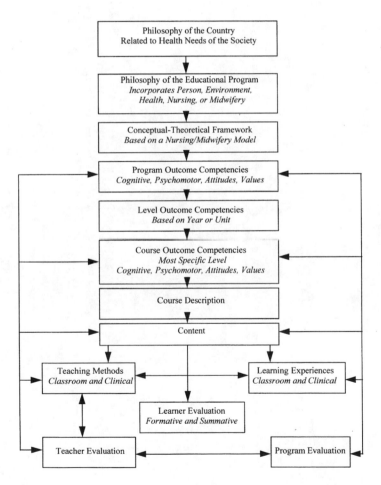

Appendix B

EVALUATING CLASSROOM TEACHING

Does the teacher

  prepare well for class?

  communicate clearly?

  use a variety of teaching methods?

  present general principles and convey conceptual understanding of material?

  clarify expectations at the beginning of class?

  promote critical thinking in learners?

  answer questions satisfactorily?

  respond helpfully to students in difficulty?

  facilitate understanding of complex situations?

  use audiovisual aids effectively?

  use distance learning technology effectively?

  encourage participation of all students?

  stimulate student interest?

  assign pertinent course readings?

  make assignments that aid in understanding course materials?

Appendix C

PEER REVIEW: EVALUATING FACULTY TEACHING/ LEADERSHIP EFFECTIVENESS

To what extent does the faculty member

transform content knowledge into pedagogically powerful ideas?

provide sound, illuminating answers to questions?

use supplemental aids that enhance learners' grasping of material?

adhere to ethical standards?

inspire inquiry and cooperative learning?

enable students to construct their own knowledge?

exhibit vision and innovation while being receptive to these same qualities in students?

exhibit enthusiasm and accomplishment?

exemplify a supportive attitude?

respect students regardless of race, culture, ethnicity, sexual preference, age, religion, or physical limitation?

give firm direction when needed?

Adapted from Ciesla, J., & Lovejoy, N. (1997). Peer review: A method for developing faculty leaders. *Nurse Educator, 22*(6), p. 41.

Appendix D

TABLE OF SPECIFICATIONS FOR CARE OF THE ESSENTIALLY NORMAL NEWBORN

Unit Outcomes	Content	Comprehension	Application	Analysis	Synthesis	Evaluation	Affective Domain	Total No. of Items	Percent of Items
Integrate a scientific knowledge base to develop and carry out a neonate management plan for the immediate physiologic adjustment to extrauterine life.	Respiratory changes.				1				
	Fetal gas exchange and hemoglobin dissociation curves effects on O2.	1				1			
	Reasons for increased pulmonary perfusion.					1			
	Implications of the adaptive process – physical and neurological.				1	1			
	Hematopoietic and renal systems.					1			
	Neonatal resuscitation.			1			1	9	18
Identify normal characteristics and deviations from the normal during the immediate and ongoing evaluation of the newborn.	Differentiate normal and abnormal findings – physical and neurological.				2				
	Normal variations in behavior according to Brazleton.	1					1		
	Considerations when examining neonates of varying ethnic backgrounds.				2				
	Interpret findings for gestational age classification.					2			
	Contraindications of commonly used medications					1		9	18
Develop a theoretical framework for maintenance of infant nutritional status.	Oral and neuromuscular development related to food intake.	1							
	Nutritional requirements and feeding guidelines for preterm, SGA, LGA.		1						
	Cultural and economic factors in feeding practices.		1				1		
	High-risk factors for alteration in nutrition.					1		5	10
Identify specific content and rationale for timing of instructions to parents for infant care.	Elimination.								
	Feeding schedules.						1		
	Cord/circumcision care.		1				1		
	Sleeping schedules.		1						
	Safety factors.					1			
	Caregiving tailored to infant behavioral characteristics.					1			
	Infant sensory stimulation.		1						
	Psychosocial adaptation.						1		
	Cultural influences to consider with parenting skills and beliefs.					1	1		

(continued)

APPENDIX D *(continued)*

Unit Outcomes	Content	Comprehension	Application	Analysis	Synthesis	Evaluation	Affective Domain	Total No. of Items	Percent of Items
	Interpretation of culturally based parenting skills that may be unsafe.					2	1		
	Danger signals to report.					1			
	Follow up care.					1	1	16	32
Explain anatomic/physiologic basis, differential diagnosis, and nurse-midwifery management, including parent counseling, for common problems of the neonate.	Vomiting.								
	Spitting up.								
	Colic.					1			
	Milk allergy.								
	Constipation.								
	Transitory diarrhea.					1			
	URI.								
	Eye discharge.								
	Thrush.					1		3	6
Analyze the problem of neonatal jaundice.	Physiology of neonatal jaundice.					1			
	Bilirubin metabolism.	1							
	Differentiate pathologic and physiologic jaundice.					1			
	Role of newborn feeding in maturation of bilirubin metabolism and excretion mechanisms.				1			4	8
Explain deviations from the normal immune response in neonates and implications for neonate health.	Cellular and humoral immunity.					1			
	Expected deficiency in immune response.				1				
	Bacterial infection -- early & late onset.	1							
	Group B strep.	1						4	8
Total Number of Items		6	6	6	14	10	8	50	
Percent of Items		12	12	12	28	20	16		100

Adapted from Linn, R. L. and Gronlund, N. E. (2000). Measurement and Assessment in Teaching (8th ed.). Englewood Cliffs, NJ: Prentice Hall.

Appendix E

SAMPLE CLINICAL SITE DATA SHEET

Site Name _____

Type of setting _____

Location _____ Date of visit _____

Miles from academic unit _____ Telephone _____

Transportation needed/available/cost _____

Type of practice _____ Hours of coverage _____

Primary contact for practice _____

Total staff (attach CV or resume for each) _____

Written policies/protocols available _____ Date ____

Medical Director if appropriate _____

Type and level of learners in setting (Who, what, how many, and when?) ____

Educational opportunities available (e.g., rounds, patient education, conferences) _____

Descriptive data on approximate number and type of patients per week/session

Procedures routinely available for learning _____

Owner at the practice _____

Continuity of care possible _____

Willingness to supervise APN/midwifery learners _____

Expectations of practice for use of clinical facility ⎯⎯⎯⎯⎯⎯⎯⎯⎯⎯⎯

Expectations of academic unit for clinical site ⎯⎯⎯⎯⎯⎯⎯⎯⎯⎯⎯⎯

Mechanisms agreed for feedback/evaluation of learner progress ⎯⎯⎯⎯⎯⎯

General impression of suitability for use as clinical site ⎯⎯⎯⎯⎯⎯⎯⎯⎯

Person(s) preparing this report ⎯⎯⎯⎯⎯⎯⎯⎯⎯⎯⎯⎯⎯⎯⎯⎯⎯⎯⎯⎯⎯⎯

Appendix F

SAMPLE CLINICAL TEACHER REPORT FORM

Learner _____ Date _____

Preceptor _____ Course/Module _____

Site _____

The following format is to be used to evaluate learner progress at set intervals (telephone contact, clinical faculty meetings, etc.).

A. *Follows Each Step of Management or Clinical Decision Making Process*

1. Collects complete data in timely manner
2. Makes correct decisions based on data collected
3. Recognizes emergency need for action (priority setting)
4. Assumes appropriate role in setting (learner, consultant, etc.)
5. Designs comprehensive plan with alternatives
6. Implements plan safely and efficiently
7. Evaluates effects of interventions appropriately

B. *Clinical Skills Development*

1. Hand skills: appropriate timing, accurate results, minimal discomfort to patient
2. Communication skills: clear, concise, complete, and accurate oral presentations to preceptor/consultant; appropriate client teaching and instructions given; legible, complete and concise written records
3. Theory base appropriate to level of learner

C. *Professional Behaviors*

    1. Accountable—responsible, dependable, and practices in accord with standards and policies; able to accurately evaluate own performance

    2. Commitment to philosophy of care of APN or midwifery discipline (patient autonomy, competence, family centered care)

    3. Demonstrates initiative and self-direction—accepts constructive criticism, new ideas and concepts, leadership potential

D. *Overall Performance Relative to Expectations (Outcomes)*

E. *Summary of Strengths and Needs*

Appendix G

SUGGESTED GUIDELINES FOR PREPARATION
OF PRECEPTORS

A. Explanation of curriculum
   1. Overall curriculum plan
      a. Philosophy and conceptual framework
      b. Terminal outcomes
      c. Plan of study—sequence of courses
         1. Core courses
         2. Clinical major courses
         3. Electives
   2. Orientation to adult learning strategies
      a. Discussion of theoretical and clinical outcomes that relate to clinical assignment
      b. Review principles of adult learning and teaching
      c. Review progress of learner to date in relation to expected clinical performance outcomes
      d. Review clinical evaluation tool and its use
B. Approach to clinical teaching
   1. Overview and introduction to clinical teaching
      a. Explore positive and negative experiences clinical instructors have had in their own teaching and learning situations
      b. Explore previous experience with teaching in clinical area (e.g., type and level of learner)
   2. Teach according to management and/or clinical decision-making process
   3. Evaluate according to the management and/or clinical decision-making process (formative and summative done during post-conference)
C. Discussion of philosophy of teaching of clinical instructor
   1. Discuss how philosophy of teaching can facilitate learning
   2. Discuss teaching techniques needed for level of learner

3. Discuss factors that promote and hinder learning in clinical site
4. Review principles of teaching and learning of particular importance in the clinical area
5. Reinforce strengths clinical instructors bring to the teaching/learning situation
6. Offer assistance as needed to refine/expand teaching expertise

D. Review of expectations of teachers and learners in the clinical area

E. Specifics of clinical instruction
1. Establish where learner is at in the beginning of his/her experience in the setting
   a. Meet with learner and review his/her progress to date in the program
   b. Review specific clinical objectives/outcomes for this rotation
   c. Revise objectives/outcomes as needed in consideration of the realities of the particular clinical site
2. Prior to each learning experience, discuss with learner his/her particular objectives for the clinical day as well as teacher expectations (pre-conference)
3. Discuss learner performance, beginning with learner self-evaluation, at the end of each clinical day (post-conference) and set learning objectives for next clinical day
4. Allow time to develop comfort and trust with learner and self as teacher
   a. Begin with close observation of learner to determine level of functioning in clinical area (novice, advanced beginner)
   b. Share rationale and expect rationale from learner, especially when the learner chooses a plan of action different from that the teacher would have chosen
   c. Select teaching method (directing, supportive, delegating) (Blanchard, 1985) appropriate to performance of learner while moving the learner toward independence of functioning
   d. Always place errors in perspective
5. Share teacher's boundaries of safety with learner
   a. Define those things the learner may do without direct teacher supervision
   b. Define those things the learner must have teacher present in order to do (at least initially)
   c. Review the practice policies and protocols of the setting

F. Review and leave written contact information for course faculty contact and encourage the clinical instructor to call with any questions or concerns

Index